GUIDE TO
CONSUMER
SERVICES

GUIDE TO
CONSUMER
SERVICES

Consumers Union's Advice On Selected Financial And Professional Services

BY THE EDITORS OF CONSUMER REPORTS
CONSUMERS UNION, MOUNT VERNON, NEW YORK

Guide to Consumer Services is a special publication of Consumers Union, the non-profit organization that publishes CONSUMER REPORTS, the monthly magazine of test reports, product Ratings, and buying guidance. Established in 1936, Consumers Union is chartered under the Not-For-Profit Corporation Law of the State of New York.

The purposes of Consumers Union, as stated in its charter, are to provide consumers with information and counsel on consumer goods and services, to give information and assistance on all matters relating to the expenditure of the family income, and to initiate and to cooperate with individual and group efforts seeking to create and maintain decent living standards.

Consumers Union derives its income solely from the sale of CONSUMER REPORTS and other publications. Consumers Union accepts no advertising and is not beholden in any way to any commercial interest. Its Ratings and reports are solely for the information and use of the readers of its publications.

Neither the Ratings nor the reports nor any other Consumers Union publications, including this book, may be used in advertising or for any commercial purpose of any nature. Consumers Union will take all steps open to it to prevent or to prosecute any such uses of its material or of its name or the name of CONSUMER REPORTS.

Contents

Introduction

CONSUMER REPORTS magazine is best known for product testing and reporting. But since its founding more than forty years ago, Consumers Union has also provided consumers with information and counsel on services as well as goods. In recent years, with consumer services accounting for more and more of the consumer dollar, CU's coverage of services has increased in scope and depth: detailed reports on health and medicine, financial guidance, how to get professional help for consumer problems. And CU monitors the consumer marketplace, the government agencies charged with its regulation, and legislation affecting consumers. Each month, two or three such reports, prepared with the same care given to CU's product-testing reports, are published in CONSUMER REPORTS.

Guide to Consumer Services is composed of a representative selection of service articles, taken from recent issues of the magazine. The reports presented here can help you make crucial decisions about health care, money matters, and shopping for services. CU guides you as income tax time comes around, before you sign an apartment lease or buy a house, when you want to deal with the landlord or to fight an unfair tax assessment. You can find out how to go about choosing a physician or dentist, shopping for credit or for shares of stock, selecting a summer camp or an auto mechanic, getting the best buy in prescription drugs or a hearing aid. Each report has been reviewed, revised, and updated to reflect the latest information available when we went to press.

A good cross-section of the services marketplace is covered in *Guide to Consumer Services*. But the field of consumer services is by no means exhausted with this book. There is a continuing need for reliable, knowledgeable, readable information about many other consumer services. For this reason, CU will continue to report regularly on consumer services—in addition to consumer products—in the pages of CONSUMER REPORTS and in other CU special publications.

THE EDITORS OF CONSUMER REPORTS

How to Shop for Credit

Consumer credit has been an American way of life since Colonial times, when farmers borrowed against their crops and bought much of their furniture on the installment plan. Modern forms of credit include credit cards and "no-bounce" checking accounts, but the basic theory of credit has remained the same over the centuries: Lenders rent money to those who need it. Money is thus a commodity, and someone who borrows, or rents, money pays for the privilege. The interest is the fee for renting money.

A prospective borrower must always remember that lenders are in the business of credit, *not* in the business of doing favors. If lenders offer inviting repayment terms, they're not doing it just to be nice; they're doing it to increase their sales volume. "Easy credit"—both with credit cards and installment loans—has been good business for lenders. In late 1976, Americans owed about $169 billion (excluding mortgages) and were using about 14 percent of their take-home pay for that debt. Although many buy on credit or borrow money, not all spend much time shopping around. Credit can be expensive (in November 1976, for example, some California banks were charging more than 16 percent for personal loans), but at some banks credit is more expensive than at others.

The money saved by borrowing from the lowest-cost lender can be considerable, especially when the loan is a large one. For example, in late 1976, one of the largest commercial banks in New York City charged 13.38 percent for a $3,000 personal loan.* A large savings bank in the same city charged 10.88 percent for the same type of loan. If you paid off the $3,000 loan over three years, you would pay the commercial bank a total of $658.32 in interest; by contrast, the loan from the savings bank would cost you only $529.20 —a savings of $129.12. (In a limited survey of loan rates in 1974, CU commonly found variations of about two percentage points among rates charged by a number of banking institutions within the same city.)

The most important thing to do when shopping for credit is to compare the *annual percentage rates* charged by different institutions. The annual percentage rate (the true annual interest rate) includes the basic finance charge plus any additional costs, such as credit investigation fees, service charges, and mandatory insurance premiums. The 1968 Truth-in-Lending laws require lenders to quote the cost of credit in terms of the annual percentage rate.

Don't take it for granted that all lenders necessarily obey the Truth-in-Lending laws—indications are otherwise. Studies have shown that some institutions do not cite annual percentage rates but instead still illegally quote "add-on" or "discount" rates to the public. Those rates, which

---

*Except where otherwise noted, all interest rates mentioned in this report are as of November 1976 and may have changed since then.

are used internally by banks, are misleading; they are equal to roughly *half* of the annual percentage rates. (Adequate enforcement of the relevant Truth-in-Lending laws has been a problem, according to government officials.)

For several years, the Federal Reserve Board has collected consumer information on individual bank loan rates across the country. The Federal Reserve's reluctance to release this information to the public has been a controversial issue. In 1973, CU sued for release of comparative loan rates under the Freedom of Information Act. As a result, consumers can now obtain a list of rate information similar to the one printed below.

COMPARISON OF LOAN RATES

Listed below are annual percentage rates on three types of consumer loans reported to the government in September 1976 by commercial banks located in fourteen large metropolitan areas. Rates may have changed since, but other bank surveys show that *relative* differences tend to remain constant.

	AUTO Ⓐ	CONSUMER GOODS Ⓑ	PERSONAL Ⓒ
BOSTON AREA			
First National Bank of Boston	11.96	12.47	14.01
National Shawmut Bank of Boston	11.52	13.80	14.01
New England Merchants National Bank	11.08	None	14.01
State Street Bank and Trust Co.	11.52	13.80	13.57
Hancock Bank & Trust Co., Quincy, Mass.	10.64	12.47	14.89
CHICAGO AREA			
Aurora National Bank, Aurora, Ill.	10.26	13.30	13.55
American National Bank and Trust Co.	10.64	12.91	12.67
Central National Bank	11.06	12.91	12.68

Ⓐ *New-automobile loans, 36 months.*
Ⓑ *Loans for TV sets, major appliances, furniture, etc., 24 months.*
Ⓒ *Unsecured personal loans, 12 months.*

11

	AUTO [A]	CONSUMER GOODS [B]	PERSONAL [C]
Continental Illinois National Bank and Trust Co.	10.50	None	11.00
First Commercial Bank	10.20	None	None
First National Bank of Chicago	11.52	12.91	12.67
Harris Trust and Savings Bank	11.08	None	12.68
La Salle National Bank	10.87	None	12.68
Main Bank of Chicago	11.79	10.90	12.68
Marquette National Bank	11.32	12.91	12.68
Merchandise National Bank of Chicago	10.20	12.91	12.67
National Security Bank of Chicago	10.20	None	12.68
Northern Trust Co.	11.08	12.91	12.68

CLEVELAND AREA

	AUTO [A]	CONSUMER GOODS [B]	PERSONAL [C]
First National Bank of Akron, Akron, Ohio	10.20	13.08	14.45
Cleveland Trust	10.64	12.91	14.45
National City Bank	11.08	14.68	14.45
Lorain City Savings and Trust Co., Elyria, Ohio	11.96	14.68	13.57
First National Bank and Trust Co. of Ravenna, Ravenna, Ohio	11.98	None	14.45

DALLAS-FORT WORTH AREA

	AUTO [A]	CONSUMER GOODS [B]	PERSONAL [C]
First National Bank in Dallas	11.08	12.91	19.72
Mercantile National Bank at Dallas	11.10	12.90	14.04
Republic National Bank of Dallas	10.20	12.02	17.97
First National Bank of Fort Worth	11.08	12.91	12.68
Fort Worth National Bank	10.20	14.24	14.45

DETROIT AREA

	AUTO [A]	CONSUMER GOODS [B]	PERSONAL [C]
Bank of the Commonwealth	12.83	12.91	12.68
City National Bank	10.20	12.91	12.67
Detroit Bank and Trust Co.	11.08	12.91	12.91
Manufacturers National Bank of Detroit	12.83	14.68	12.68
Michigan National Bank of Detroit	11.08	12.02	11.79
National Bank of Detroit	12.25	None	17.10
First National Bank in Mount Clemens, Mich.	11.08	12.91	12.68
Community National Bank of Pontiac, Mich.	11.08	13.57	14.00
Warren Bank, Warren, Mich.	10.76	13.89	15.57

[A] *New-automobile loans, 36 months.*
[B] *Loans for TV sets, major appliances, furniture, etc., 24 months.*
[C] *Unsecured personal loans, 12 months.*

	AUTO Ⓐ	CONSUMER GOODS Ⓑ	PERSONAL Ⓒ
LOS ANGELES AREA			
Valley National Bank, Glendale, Calif.	10.64	10.58	10.00
Union Bank	11.52	None	13.57
United California Bank	12.00	None	15.00
MIAMI AREA			
Florida National Bank at Coral Gables, Fla.	10.34	None	14.22
Century National Bank of Coral Ridge, Fort Lauderdale, Fla.	10.00	None	13.87
Century National Bank of Broward, Fort Lauderdale, Fla.	10.00	11.50	11.50
Fort Lauderdale National Bank, Fort Lauderdale, Fla.	None	14.92	13.91
City National Bank of Miami	11.00	11.13	None
NEW YORK CITY AREA			
National Community Bank of Rutherford, N.J.	11.18	11.37	11.58
Bankers Trust Co.	13.38	12.59	11.58
Bank of New York	12.13	12.59	11.58
Chase Manhattan Bank	13.38	12.59	11.58
Chemical Bank	13.38	12.59	11.58
First National City Bank	13.38	None	11.58
Irving Trust Co.	13.38	None	11.58
National Bank of North America	13.38	12.59	11.58
Chemical Bank Hudson Valley, Nyack, N.Y.	10.87	12.58	11.57
Scarsdale National Bank and Trust Co., Scarsdale, N.Y.	10.27	12.59	11.58
National Bank of Westchester, White Plains, N.Y.	10.00	11.50	11.50
NEWARK, N.J., AREA			
Maplewood Bank and Trust Co., Maplewood, N.J.	10.88	11.37	11.58
Fidelity Union Trust Co.	11.80	None	11.58
First National State Bank of New Jersey	11.18	None	9.00
Midlantic National Bank	11.18	None	11.58
First National Bank of Central Jersey, Somerville, N.J.	11.18	None	11.58
Summit and Elizabeth Trust Co., Summit, N.J.	11.08	11.57	11.34
Union Center National Bank, Union, N.J.	9.25	11.00	11.00

13

	AUTO Ⓐ	CONSUMER GOODS Ⓑ	PERSONAL Ⓒ
PHILADELPHIA AREA			
Bank of New Jersey, Camden, N.J.	10.20	11.37	11.58
Central Penn National Bank, Bala-Cynwyd, Pa.	10.07	None	11.53
First Pennsylvania Banking and Trust Co., Bala-Cynwyd, Pa.	10.20	None	11.58
Girard Trust Bank, Bala-Cynwyd, Pa.	11.08	None	12.43
Fidelity Bank, Rosemont, Pa.	9.76	None	12.00
PITTSBURGH AREA			
Pittsburgh National Bank, Jeannette, Pa.	10.64	12.58	11.57
Equibank	11.08	14.68	10.90
Mellon Bank	10.91	12.45	11.48
Union National Bank of Pittsburgh	10.96	14.57	11.54
First National Bank and Trust Co., Washington, Pa.	11.08	12.59	11.58
SAN FRANCISCO AREA			
Bank of California	10.20	13.79	13.79
Bank of America National Trust and Savings Association	11.52	None	13.57
Crocker National Bank	12.50	15.50	15.50
Wells Fargo Bank	12.67	15.46	15.46
SEATTLE AREA			
Pacific National Bank of Washington	10.00	12.00	12.00
Peoples National Bank of Washington	10.50	12.00	12.00
Rainier National Bank	12.00	12.00	12.00
Seattle First National Bank	10.50	12.00	12.00
WASHINGTON, D.C., AREA			
American Security and Trust Co.	9.00	None	11.00
Madison National Bank	10.00	11.50	11.50
National Bank of Washington	10.00	11.50	11.50
National Savings and Trust Co.	9.50	11.50	None
Riggs National Bank of Washington, D.C.	10.00	11.00	11.00
Security National Bank	10.00	11.50	11.50
United Virginia Bank, Vienna, Va.	10.20	12.91	12.68

Ⓐ *New-automobile loans, 36 months.*
Ⓑ *Loans for TV sets, major appliances, furniture, etc., 24 months.*
Ⓒ *Unsecured personal loans, 12 months.*

The listing may not include your bank, but it should give you an idea of comparative rates in your area. To obtain the most current survey, write (or telephone) the Freedom of Information Office, Federal Reserve Board, Washington, D.C. 20551. Or get in touch with the vice-president in charge of public relations at one of the Federal Reserve's twelve district banks.* Be sure to specify the geographic area for which you want the information. Of course, things would be much easier if local banks would post their rates. In 1975, CU petitioned the Federal Reserve to require such posting, but the Board has not yet acted on the petition.

Banks do tend to publicize all kinds of nonmonetary factors—friendly credit officers, simplified loan application forms, "instant" loans approved over the phone—and this further complicates credit shopping. Ignore such advertising smoke screens; look for the lowest annual percentage rate and the type of credit that best meets your needs. This report will help you to do that. It concentrates on the kinds of credit offered by commercial banks, mutual savings banks, and savings and loan associations, and also describes some alternative sources of credit.

OPEN-END CREDIT

With open-end credit (also called revolving credit), which includes bank credit cards and most department-store charge accounts, consumers in most cases have the option of paying the entire amount of a bill or just a part (the minimum payment amount—or more, if they wish). Because the minimum payment amount is a small part of the

*In Atlanta, Boston, Chicago, Cleveland, Dallas, Kansas City, Mo., Minneapolis, New York, Philadelphia, Richmond, St. Louis, and San Francisco.

total, a loan can be stretched out for months.

There are now on average more than two credit cards for every person in the country. Bank credit cards, such as Master Charge and BankAmericard, account for about 20 percent of all the cards in circulation. (There are also travel and entertainment cards, those issued by retail stores, and those issued by oil companies.) Credit cards usually permit a consumer to make as many purchases (or take out loans) as desired up to the maximum dollar limit, or "line" of credit, set for that particular person. Additional credit, up to the same limit, is extended as the borrower pays off the original balance. (Credit with cards such as American Express, Diner's Club, and Carte Blanche does not work this way. With these cards, the borrower must generally pay the total amount of a bill each month.)

Most banks issue bank credit cards themselves at no charge. But they often peddle the cards, too, as part of expensive package accounts. Under these plans, you pay a flat fee of about $2 to $4 per month in exchange for a variety of services—including such things as unlimited checking and lower loan rates. Since bank credit cards alone are commonly available without charge, you should be able to find one you don't have to pay for.

Banks make money from their credit cards by collecting processing fees, known as "discounts," ranging from 1 to 6 percent, from merchants who allow customers to buy goods with these cards. Banks and retailers collect monthly finance charges from customers who elect not to pay their bills in full by the due date. Indeed, they make it easy for consumers who use the cards to postpone payment for purchases. That's good business for them because of the finance charges they collect on unpaid balances. But it's bad for consumers, who needn't incur *any* finance charge if they pay their credit card bills promptly. Depending on the point in a bank's or retailer's billing cycle when one makes a transaction, thirty to sixty days may elapse before a person has to pay for a purchase. If the bill is paid during this "free ride" period, no finance charge is assessed. If the bill or a certain portion of it is *not* paid by the end of the initial billing period, however, a finance charge of 1.5 percent per month (equal to an annual percentage rate of 18 percent) is typically levied on the unpaid balance. This charge is often reduced to 1 percent per month (equal to an annual percentage rate of 12 percent) on that part of the balance above a certain limit, generally $500. (Laws in some states prohibit the annual percentage rate from going above 12 or 15 percent on revolving credit, regardless of the amount owed.)

Smart consumers use the free ride period to get the equivalent of interest-free short-term loans. They pay their bills *before* banks impose a finance charge. But banks are beginning to have second thoughts about the free ride as well as their other billing methods. Some have introduced special billing procedures for those who do not pay off their total balance by the due date. These banks now institute finance charges from the date each purchase is posted to an account, rather than from the billing date (which is usually sometime *after* the posting date). Citibank, the largest bank in New York City and second largest in the country, has abolished the free ride altogether. Its Master Charge customers who pay their bills in full before the billing date are charged a fifty-cent monthly fee anyway. In this way, it seems, the bank tries to compensate for the interest it would have earned had consumers been less conscientious.

On the other hand, one small but innovative bank, Consumers Savings Bank in Worcester, Mass., actually rewards Massachusetts consumers who use its card. It gives these customers a 1 percent rebate on the price of every item purchased with its BankAmericard and deposits the rebate in a savings account at the bank. Bank officials say the rebate operates as an incentive to customers to use the credit card more often and in this way produces more income for the bank. Out-of-state applicants had been accepted too, but the bank was so swamped that, as of this writing, out-of-staters were not being accepted.

Calculating Finance Charges

Finance charges for credit cards are not negotiable. But the amount of interest can vary greatly, depending on how the bank or retailer calculates the charges. Here are three methods in common use: The *adjusted balance method* (sometimes called the closing balance method) is the cheapest for consumers. The finance charge is calculated on the unpaid balance of the previous month, less credits and payments made in the current month. The *average daily balance method* is considerably more costly than the adjusted balance method. With this approach, the finance charges are determined by dividing the sum of the balances outstanding for each day of the billing period by the number of days in the period and then multiplying by the daily rate of interest. The longer you defer payment, the higher your average daily balance and the higher the resulting finance costs. The average daily balance method is used by most banks. The *previous balance method* can also be costly for consumers. The finance charges are calculated on the amount owed on the final billing date of the previous month. This method does not take into account any payments made to reduce the balance or any credits for returned merchandise. It is the method traditionally used by many retailers.

Some Credit Card Problems

Credit card billing can create certain problems you should be aware of.

Delayed billing. There was a time when billing statements were sometimes sent so late they arrived after the due date, making it impossible for consumers to avoid a finance charge. The problem was largely eliminated in 1975 by the Fair Credit Billing Act, which requires creditors to mail statements at least fourteen days in advance of the due date. It also requires them to acknowledge billing inquiries within thirty days and to settle complaints within ninety days. If it turns out that creditors made a mistake in billing, you do not have to pay finance charges on the disputed amount.

Billing disputes. Under the Fair Credit Billing Act, creditors must notify a consumer before issuing an unfavorable credit report on a disputed account. They are prohibited from sending dunning letters until they have acknowledged the consumer's complaints and they must specify on the monthly bill the address for correspondence on a billing dispute. If your problem is with a bank credit card bill and that problem is not cleared up, complain to the Director of the Office of Saver and Consumer Affairs, Federal Reserve Board, Washington, D.C. 20551. You may also register your complaint with the Federal Reserve Bank for the district in which the bank is located. Be sure to describe the bank practice or action objected to and to give the name and address of the bank concerned as well as your own.

Misleading numbers. When you finally do get your bill, you may be misled about the amount of money you owe. The statements of some banks (and other creditors as well) focus attention on the *minimum* amount due rather than the total owed. Of course, the more you leave unpaid, the more interest you owe. If you plan to pay the complete bill, scrutinize your statement carefully for the total amount owed. Otherwise you may be surprised to find a finance charge on your next statement.

Vague reporting of transactions. Many banks and department stores have abandoned so-called country club billing, which provides the customer with copies of each charge slip along with the monthly bill. They've turned instead to "descriptive" billing. By simply listing the charge transactions made the previous month, bankers and retailers cut down on their paperwork and so save money. The trouble with descriptive billing is that it often isn't very descriptive. The problem is worse in the case of bank credit card bills if the merchant's name is that of a parent company, not the name of the firm with which you actually conducted your business. What's more, the date on the bill may be the date the transaction was posted to your account, not the date of purchase. Being billed by unfamiliar sellers on dates when you did not shop can be very confusing. If your bank or department store uses descriptive billing, save your purchase receipts. They will be your only complete record of purchase and might help you to decipher your statement.

Defective merchandise. What happens if the product you purchase on credit turns out to be defective? It used to be that customers had to pay the bill anyway or risk legal retribution. But an important section of the Fair Credit Billing Act gives credit card holders the right to withhold payment for defective items costing more than $50. Unfortunately, this applies only to purchases made in the buyer's home state or within a hundred miles of the place the card was issued.

When it comes to defective credit purchases that are financed on installment contracts from a third party (for example, third-party contracts to finance automobiles, furniture, or other major purchases), the Federal Trade Commission (FTC) has ruled that a consumer has the right to defend nonpayment of a purchase and to raise claims against the credit company itself, not just the merchant.

Little Loans—Big Charges

Banks have found various ways to enable you to use your bank credit card to get "instant" loans. Here are two.

Cash advances. Banks allow credit card customers to obtain small loans through a device known as the "cash advance." To get the cash, you simply present your credit card at the bank, fill out a form indicating the amount of money desired (it must fall within your permissible line of credit), and give the form to a teller. Banks have made the process so simple that you almost feel the money belongs to you. But the cost of such "painless" loans can be quite high. In California, for instance, the price can be as high as 1.5 percent per month, or an annual percentage rate of 18 percent. And some banks assess an additional "transaction fee" for processing the loan. Such a fee, coupled with a basic annual percentage rate of 18 percent, can result in an interest cost far above that for installment loans (see pages 24-29) at many of these same banks. In addition, interest on a cash advance, unlike interest on most credit card purchases, begins from the date the transaction is made. There is no free-ride period.

It costs a bank about $7.50 to process a cash advance, about $50 to process an installment loan. And so a number of large banks now refuse to make installment loans for amounts under $1,000 or $2,000. This means that if you want to borrow less than the bank's minimum for an installment loan, you may wish to get the money as a cash advance. It's good business for banks to make loans that cost them less, but a cash advance may well cost you more. If you find yourself in this situation, it may be worthwhile for you to check with other banks to see if you can get an installment loan for the amount you need at an interest rate below that for a cash advance.

Blank checks. Some banks also issue blank "checks" that can be used as cash advances. The banks will often stress the versatility of these blank checks, suggesting that they can be used like regular checks to pay doctors, tax collectors, and others who don't accept credit cards. But there are finance charges for using the checks. Banks were not always forthright about telling their customers about these charges. In 1975, therefore, the Federal Reserve Board passed a Truth-in-Lending regulation requiring creditors to disclose the charges very clearly.

No-Bounce Checking

The latest gimmick in open-end credit is No-Bounce Checking, which also goes by such names as Overdraft Checking, Privilege Checking, and Checking Plus. With such an account, you are granted a prearranged line of credit and can overdraw your checking account up to that amount without the checks bouncing. The overdraft is treated as a loan, and interest is charged on it.

One way that bankers maximize income on this type of credit is by advancing customers more money than is actually needed to cover an overdraft. Many banks insist that advances be in multiples of $50 or $100, regardless of the amount of the overdraft. The result: You could overdraw your account by only one dollar and be charged for a hundred-dollar loan. Some banks do, however, advance the exact amount of the overdraft. We suggest you look for them. When you're ready to repay an overdraft, some banks require you to use special deposit slips for loan repayment. Other banks automatically credit money deposited in a checking account as payment toward the overdraft loan. The latter method is the preferable one because it's less cumbersome for consumers. What's more, it avoids the misunderstanding common with the first method: thinking that routine deposits get rid of the debt.

Overdraft checking can be useful occasionally as protection against unforeseen expenses. In such cases it can eliminate the embarrassment of a bounced check—and it may even cost less than a bounced check. But it's unwise to use overdrafts routinely. The interest rates on overdraft loans generally range from 1 to 1.5 percent per month —equal to an annual percentage rate of 12 to 18 percent.

If you have a no-bounce checking account and want to close it, be sure to notify the bank in writing. Some consumers who left a small balance in their unused account — expecting service fees eventually to deplete the account to zero—discovered that the accumulated service fees not only exhausted the balance but triggered an unwelcome overdraft loan as well.

Try to Pay on Time

The open-end credit provided by bank and most department store credit cards, cash advances, and overdraft checking can be useful and convenient so long as you understand it will cost you money whenever you don't pay the bill quickly and in full. It takes self-discipline to keep your purchases within the limits of your income, enjoy the thirty-to-sixty-day free ride on a credit card, and then pay up before any finance charge is assessed. But consider the following incentives to pay promptly:

Finance charge. Assume you typically have an average daily balance of $500 in purchases outstanding on your credit card. If you regularly fail to pay in full by the due date (and about two-thirds of Americans do fail), that balance would be subject to a finance charge equal to an annual percentage rate of 18 percent and could result in an interest bill of at least $90 over a year's time.

Interest on interest. Banks and department stores compound, or charge interest on, interest. The interest assessed on your unpaid balance each month becomes part of the balance against which interest is charged the following month. Say you have an unpaid balance of $100 and you make no payment. The monthly interest charge of 1.5 percent adds $1.50 to that sum. The following month, the interest charge is figured on $101.50, not $100.

Late charges. Failure to pay the minimum amount due each month sometimes triggers late charges, which can be substantial over a year's time. As a general rule, these charges amount to 5 percent of the minimum monthly payment, up to a maximum of $5. The charges are also added to the unpaid balance and become part of the base on which interest is figured in the next month's accounting.

If you can't manage to pay your credit card bills fully within a fairly short period—six months at the most—CU suggests you stop using credit cards and other forms of revolving credit. Instead, get an installment loan from your bank or from one of the cheaper credit sources we'll discuss later in this report.

CLOSED-END CREDIT

With closed-end credit—which is also called installment credit—a specific amount is borrowed for, and repaid during, a specific time period. Payments are usually made in equal monthly installments. Installment credit is the means by which many Americans finance such major purchases as automobiles, furniture, and major appliances. You may be under the impression that all banks charge pretty much the same rates for such loans, but in fact rates vary widely. Always shop for the lowest rate before giving an institution your credit business.

In our limited study of loan rates in 1974, CU found significant differences between large and small banks. With new-car loans, for instance, the small banks charged an average annual percentage rate of about 10 percent, whereas the large banks charged an average annual percentage rate of 11.5 percent. But there were exceptions. Not all small banks offered the cheapest installment loans, and the small banks that did charge low rates on one type of loan didn't necessarily charge the lowest rates on other types. (See the listing on pages 11-14 for selected, more recent interest rates available from the Federal Reserve Board.)

In shopping for an installment loan, *don't hesitate to bargain for a lower price.* Banks like to give the impression that their loan charges are inflexible, but banks often have a range of permissible rates. Most of the commercial banks that participated in our survey indicated that their rates were indeed negotiable. A CU shopper was able to negotiate, with no trouble at all, a reduction of a full percentage point on a personal loan rate. An interesting note: As the shopper prepared to leave, the credit officer commented, "That's the first time a customer ever asked about a lower rate. Usually they just ask about the monthly payments."

Traditionally, installment loans (with the exception of mortgages) have been the province of commercial banks because savings institutions have been prohibited from entering this field. But the legal restraints are beginning to ease and mutual savings banks and savings and loan associations in some states can now offer certain kinds of installment loans. According to CU's 1974 banking survey, the rates for these installment loans are often lower than the rates charged by commercial banks.

What Affects Interest Rates?

There are a number of considerations that can affect the interest rate charged on a loan. One is the credit standing of the borrower. To measure this, banks traditionally have used a formula known as the three Cs of credit—character, capacity, and collateral.

Character is measured by such things as continuous employment in the same line of work for a number of years and residence in the same area for a certain length of time. Capacity is measured by a level of income sufficient to pay off the loan plus any other debts that may be outstanding. Collateral is measured by a potential borrower's assets, such as a car, a house, savings, and securities. (Some institutions red-flag persons in certain occupations as potential credit risks. Among those considered credit risks are beauticians, bartenders, foreign diplomats, dock workers, noncommissioned military personnel, taxi drivers, and freelance artists, writers, and musicians.)

A second factor affecting the interest rate is the amount of money borrowed. Generally, the larger the loan, the lower the rate. On a personal loan, for instance, a bank may have one rate if the loan is for less than $1,000, another rate if it is between $1,000 and $3,000, and a third rate if it is for more than $3,000.

A third consideration in determining the interest rate is the type of loan. Traditionally, new-car loans carry relatively low rates because the car represents collateral—the lender can repossess the car and sell it if the borrower defaults. By contrast, unsecured personal loans (loans that are not backed by collateral) are more expensive. There are also specialized loans to finance such things as home improvement or college tuition. The rates on those fall somewhere between new-car loans and unsecured personal loans.

The Cheapest Ways to Borrow

The most economical way to borrow is to borrow against accumulated assets, which may be in the form of a savings account or in the form of stocks and bonds. Loans backed by such assets usually carry lower annual percentage rates than those on other types of loans. How much lower depends on the type of collateral you put up.

Savings institutions specialize in loans backed by savings accounts. With such loans, called passbook loans, you can usually borrow against 90 percent or more of the money in your savings account. Many banks—about three-quarters, according to our 1974 survey—let you use your savings account progressively as you pay off your loan. With the others you cannot touch any of your savings until you've repaid your entire loan, an unnecessarily harsh rule.

The interest rates on passbook loans are often the lowest available from banking institutions. In late 1976, for instance, a CU shopper found that the largest savings bank in New York (and the country), the Bowery Savings Bank, charged an annual percentage rate of 8 percent on a regular passbook loan, whereas the largest commercial banks in the city charged about 3½ percentage points more.

The interest rate on loans against securities may not be as low as those against savings accounts and you may not be able to get as large a loan as you need. The amount that can be borrowed from banks against stocks and bonds is regulated by the federal government. Sometimes it's about half the current value of the securities; sometimes more, sometimes less. Moreover, if the value of the securities suddenly drops below the bank's limit, you may have to prepay part of the loan (i.e., pay it off early) or put up more collateral.

Installment Loan Mathematics

Although all lenders are required to quote finance charges in terms of the annual percentage rate, they can use different methods, such as the add-on or the discount method, which we mentioned earlier, to calculate them. These charges are then converted into the equivalent annual percentage rates—a procedure followed by most banks.

But a number of banks have adopted the *simple interest* method. Under this approach a bank charges interest only on the exact amount borrowed for the exact length of time it is loaned. This method in effect rewards you for paying early and automatically increases your finance charges the longer you take to pay.

A regular repayment schedule with equal monthly payments is usually set up, with a final "equalizer" payment at the end. If you follow the repayment schedule exactly, your final payment will be approximately the same size as all the previous ones. But if you are regularly late, the final payment will be a little larger, because you will have had use of the money longer than with the add-on or discount method. (One would think that a bank using the simple interest rate would not also bill you for late charges since you've already paid more in finance charges because you've taken longer to pay. But some banks do.) Similarly, if you consistently make payments ahead of time, your final payment will be somewhat smaller than the payments that were made earlier.

Among lenders charging the same annual percentage rate, choose the one that calculates the rate using the simple interest method (ask the loan officer about it) without a late charge. If you find only rates figured with the add-on or discount method, you need still more information—the annual percentage rate.

Creditors that use the add-on or discount method to figure finance charges also use one of two methods to determine how much interest you get back if you repay a loan early. These are the actuarial method and the so-called Rule of 78's. You needn't learn how they work, but you should know this: Given the same annual percentage rates, favor the bank that uses the actuarial method, especially if you are borrowing fairly large sums of money over fairly long periods—say $10,000 over four years. The difference between the two methods is inconsequential when the amount borrowed is smaller and for a shorter period—say $2,000 for two years.

Credit Life Insurance

Most people take out credit life insurance when they borrow. This covers repayment of a loan should the borrower die. The practice of including insurance premiums along with loan payments has been widely criticized by government regulators. They claim consumers are railroaded into purchasing the insurance at inflated prices. The Truth-in-Lending laws say that the insurance costs must be reflected both in the quoted finance charge and in the annual percentage rate—unless the insurance is an option the borrower may refuse.

The FTC and consumer groups have done studies to determine just how optional the purchase of credit life insurance is. In 1975, trade figures showed that in some states 95 percent of the persons borrowing from consumer finance companies had purchased credit life insurance, a figure authorities consider to be remarkably high. The Federal Reserve Board has also investigated the problem and recommended to Congress that Truth-in-Lending laws be amended to establish a period of time after the purchase of insurance for borrowers to cancel if they so desire.

Banks and finance companies push credit life insurance because they profit from commissions based on the size of the premiums; the higher the premium, the larger the commission. But the question is, does a borrower *need* the insurance? Answer: If you have enough life insurance to protect your family *and* repay the debt, you don't need more. If not, credit life insurance might be worth buying —or you may want to reconsider your personal insurance program.

Repayment Problems

Nobody likes to think about it when applying for a loan, but circumstances may force a borrower to fall behind on payments. If that happens to you, contact your creditors immediately to explain the situation. In doing so you will demonstrate a sense of responsibility and may prevent harsh legal action. If your loan and your savings or checking accounts are with the same bank, the bank is permitted to seize money from your account without prior notice or court hearing, but generally banks do so only as a last resort and when loan payments are long overdue. If your bank is particularly intransigent, however, you may want to prevent a recurrence by transferring your account to an institution that does not hold your loan.

Should you run into credit problems, you may wish to refer to a nonprofit credit counseling center. (As of this writing, there are 216 such centers in the United States.)

The centers help set up, at no charge, realistic budgets for people burdened by debt. They also intercede with creditors so that borrowers trying to repay their debts are not harassed. You can get a list of the centers by writing to the National Foundation for Consumer Credit, 1819 H Street, Washington, D.C. 20006. Other possible sources of help with budgeting are local family and child service organizations set up by county and city governments. Many of these organizations provide free budget counseling as part of their overall family assistance programs.

Beware of "consolidation" loans, which lenders push as the low-cost answer to all debt difficulties. Consolidation loans may create more problems than they resolve. Bankruptcy is a last resort, but in some circumstances it may be the only sensible solution. You'd be well advised to seek financial counseling, including possible legal assistance (for example, from the Legal Aid Society), before you decide to proceed with either a consolidation loan or bankruptcy.

Discrimination at the Credit Window

For many people, a discussion of how to shop for credit is irrelevant because they can't get a loan at any price. Many of these people are nonwhite, women, or older people. Discrimination, which exists in other industries, is no stranger to financial circles. A 1972 study by the Council on Economic Priorities found it "endemic to commercial banking" and maintained it was "perpetuated by federal law, policy, and complacency." In 1974, the United States Commission on Civil Rights surveyed mortgage-lending practices in Hartford, Conn., and discovered such widespread discrimination that it called the system "a stacked deck."

Such reports finally prompted Congress to pass the

Equal Credit Opportunity Act, which became law in October 1975. The act bars lenders from discriminating against borrowers on the basis of sex or marital status. Amendments to the act also prohibit credit discrimination based on race, color, religion, national origin, age, receipt of income from public assistance programs, and good faith exercise of rights under other consumer protection laws, such as Fair Credit Billing and Truth-in-Lending. The amendments will become effective in mid-1977. Covered by Equal Credit Opportunity are all personal and commercial credit transactions including cash loans, installment sales, mortgage loans, and revolving charge accounts. Unfortunately, just as there continue to be violations of Truth-in-Lending statutes, as we noted earlier, so may there be some violations of the Equal Credit Opportunity law.

If you are turned down for credit, you should always try to find out the reason why. The reason may be that a creditor received adverse information about you from a credit bureau.

Under the Fair Credit Reporting Act, if you are rejected for credit because of a credit bureau report, the institution that turns you down must give you the name and address of the bureau. Upon request and proper identification, the credit bureau must tell you "the nature and substance of all information" in its file about you, except medical information, and must give you the source. (You do not have the right to see the files or to know the sources of hearsay evidence about your character, reputation, and personal life.) The credit bureau must tell you the firms that received your credit record during the preceding six months. The credit bureau must reinvestigate information that you say is incorrect or incomplete and must promptly correct any inaccurate data and delete any unverifiable data. At your specific request, it must send notice of the correction to all who received your report in the previous six months. If the dispute cannot be settled by investigation, you may put in the file a statement of up to one hundred words giving your side of the argument, and the bureau must include your statement in any future report. At your request, the bureau must also send copies of your statement to those who have received the disputed information. The credit bureau must not charge you for any of those services if you write the bureau within thirty days of official notice of the issuance of a bad credit report about you.

If you suspect you have been rejected because of your race, age, or sex rather than because of your financial condition, you should complain. Write a letter to the institution that turned you down and be sure to send a copy of the letter to the Director of the Office of Saver and Consumer Affairs of the Federal Reserve Board, Washington, D.C. 20551.

A woman who is married and who works should bear in mind the possibility that divorce or widowhood may one day make it necessary for her to obtain credit as an individual. Or a woman may wish to borrow as an individual now.

In order to qualify for credit, it's necessary to establish a financial identity. You establish a financial identity by maintaining your own checking and savings accounts and by obtaining credit cards in your own name. Since some banks do not feel that faithful payment of credit card bills provides enough evidence of how a person will handle a mortgage, a woman might also consider taking out and repaying a small installment loan to create the necessary credit history. The borrowed money can be deposited in a savings account, where the interest it earns will help offset the cost of the loan.

OTHER SOURCES OF CREDIT

So far, we've talked about the types of credit you can obtain directly from banking institutions. But consumers can obtain credit from other sources. Some offer it at rates much lower than banks and others at rates much higher. Here are four major alternative sources of financing.

Credit unions. Credit unions are nonprofit savings-and-borrowing organizations that are owned and run by their depositors, who generally have a common tie, such as the same employer. There are some twenty-three thousand credit unions in the country; about two-thirds are federally insured for up to $40,000 per account (state insurance protects some of the other credit unions). The annual percentage rates charged by these nonprofit organizations generally start at about 9 percent and may not go above 12 percent. An analysis in mid-1976 by the National Credit Union Administration, which regulates federally chartered credit unions, found that credit union rates were consistently and significantly lower than those of commercial banks and finance companies for all classes of consumer loans. Credit unions undercut commercial banks by only four-tenths of a percentage point on automobile loans but by more than a full percentage point on personal loans and loans for consumer goods.

Credit life insurance is often included in these rates and is not reflected as an additional charge, as it is with some banks. There are also no prepayment penalties, and some well-established credit unions also refund a portion of the interest paid by their borrowing members after the yearly books are balanced. Such refunds can reduce the cost of a loan to well below the contractual rate.

However, many credit unions insist on wage assignments. Such assignments allow a credit union to deduct loan payments from the salaries of delinquent borrowers without court hearings.

A few states, including New York, permit *open-charter* credit unions, which any resident of the state may join. To learn more about credit unions, contact your state credit union league (usually listed in phone directories under the state's name) or you can write to the Credit Union National Association, Box 431, 1617 Sherman Avenue, Madison, Wis. 53701.

Life insurance companies. CU believes that "term" life insurance is the most economical type of insurance for the needs of most people. If you have already purchased the more expensive "whole life" insurance, however, your policy can serve as collateral for some of the cheapest loans around. Under the terms of most whole-life contracts, a policyholder is entitled to borrow most or all of the accumulated cash value of the policy at a guaranteed rate. The rate on most new policies being written today ranges from 6 to 8 percent, and in New York State, the rate is limited to 5 percent. The loans can usually be made with a minimum of red tape and technically don't even have to be repaid. But note this well: Borrowing against a life insurance policy reduces the financial protection for the policy's beneficiaries, and financial protection is an insurance policy's only good reason for being.

Automobile dealers and other retailers. Automobile dealers usually offer to finance new or used cars. Such loans are invariably expensive—usually about two percentage points above a typical bank installment loan used to finance new cars. True, an automobile dealer will make things convenient: There's a minimum of paperwork and of credit investigation since the dealers want to sell their cars and figure speedy loans will help them do it. One way or another, however, the source of such credit is a bank. If *you* go to a bank instead of letting the dealer fetch the money for you, you can often save $100 or more in financing costs. The same advice holds true for installment credit offered by other retailers, whether they're selling furniture or television sets. You're always better off getting your loan directly from the source of the money.

Finance companies. These firms, which include companies like Household Finance and Beneficial Finance, are usually the most expensive legal sources of loans. In most states, the annual percentage rates they charge on small loans (under $300) will range from 30 to 36 percent; the rates typically decline to about 21 percent on larger loans (roughly $1,200 to $3,000). Finance companies usually lend to low-income, high-risk borrowers of small sums (persons whom banks most often turn away). They also compete with banks for high-income, high risk borrowers. Finance companies' rates thus reflect the characteristics of their customers. Don't go to a finance company unless you've tried to get a loan from a bank, savings institution, or a credit union.

RECOMMENDATIONS

Use credit with care. Here's a rule of thumb: Keep your debt payments (excluding mortgage payments) to no more than 20 percent of your take-home pay and limit them to 15 percent if you can. Interest rates have risen so steeply that the average consumer may pay $15 or more for every $100 borrowed. (There are some tax advantages to borrowing, but they are primarily for persons in extremely high tax brackets who can take advantage of tax loopholes through complex credit transactions. For the average American, the cost of borrowing money has little if any off-setting tax value.)

Credit cards can make life easy so long as you know how to use them. Get cards from banks that issue them free. Try to pay your bills promptly, preferably in that thirty-to-sixty-day, free-ride period before a finance charge is levied. Avoid a bank that charges a service fee if you pay promptly. If you let your repayments stretch out beyond six months, you're probably better off with an installment loan, especially when the amounts involved are substantial—$500 or more.

Automatic overdraft privileges are convenient, but they may very well be expensive if used routinely. Use the privilege only in emergencies. Look for banks that permit overdrafts for the exact amount needed rather than in multiples of $50 or $100. Choose banks that allow you to repay your overdrafts automatically, through deposits in your checking account. Discipline yourself to liquidate such debts as quickly as possible—within six months at the most. Otherwise, once again, you'd be better off with an installment loan.

If you choose an installment loan, look for the cheapest source possible—the one with the lowest annual percentage rate. If you have already purchased an expensive whole-life insurance policy and there is sufficient cash value, you may decide to start with your insurance company. Otherwise, begin with a credit union, if you belong to one, and compare the rates it offers to those charged by a number of banks and savings institutions in your area. Look for an institution that uses the simple interest method and does not assess late charges. Resist attempts to make you agree to wage garnishment provisions as a condition for obtaining the loan.

Income Taxes

WHERE TO GO FOR TAX HELP

The Commissioner of the Internal Revenue Service (IRS) maintains that most persons should be able to prepare their own tax returns. But his fellow citizens obviously don't share his optimism. In 1976, Americans probably spent more than $1 billion to have someone else make out their tax forms. At least half, and perhaps as many as 70 percent, of the eighty million or so individual returns filed were prepared by someone other than the taxpayer.

The reason: an incredibly complicated tax code and regulations that, together, run to some six thousand pages of fine print whose meaning is often open to differing interpretations. The law is so complex that a government study found you need a college education simply to understand the instructions for claiming certain itemized deductions.

Complexity and ambiguity inevitably lead to error. After auditing a random sample of tax returns for 1969, the IRS estimated that about half of all returns filed that year contained mistakes. A selected survey of a group of returns filed in 1971 indicated that two-thirds of them were incorrect. A return was most likely to be accurate when it was prepared by the individual taxpayer, the IRS, or the most highly skilled (and most expensive) accountant.

An innocent error on a return might result in your paying more taxes than you owe—or less. If the IRS decides your underestimation is serious enough, the likelihood of your being audited increases. Generally, an audit doesn't take place for at least six months after a return is filed and can take place up to three years afterward. The time involved in reconstituting old records and visiting the IRS office for the examination, plus the mental anguish of the whole procedure, may well make you wish you'd exerted a more careful watch over the preparation of your return in the first place.

This report will examine the seven main sources of help open to taxpayers.

1. Helping yourself. An intelligent do-it-yourself approach is cheap—all it takes are a few IRS publications, commercial guides, time, and perhaps a calculator. Some people even consider it fun.

2. Help from the IRS. Under certain conditions, the IRS will compute your tax by mail or help you to do it yourself at an IRS office.

3. Help from a local tax service, often individuals who operate out of storefronts and close up shop after tax season.

4. Help from a national tax service, such as H & R Block, which keeps skeleton offices open throughout the year.

5. Help from an "enrolled agent," a person who has passed a government examination but need not meet any educational requirements.

6. Help from a "public accountant," a person who does accounting work but who, in most states, needn't meet any educational requirements nor pass a special examination.

7. **Help from a "certified public accountant,"** or CPA. CPAs are usually college graduates who have passed a rigorous examination in accounting.

1. Helping Yourself

Most taxpayers lead relatively simple economic lives. If you're among that majority, you should be able to figure your own taxes accurately, especially if you have access to a calculator or an adding machine.

What's a "simple" economic life? The experts say it's one where the annual income is under $25,000 or $30,000 and comes from no sources other than wages, salary, tips, interest, dividends, and pensions. Income from other sources, such as rental property or a business, generally introduces enough tax complexity to warrant professional help.

The first step in preparing your own return is to set up a checklist for income and deductions. The instruction booklet for the long form, 1040, is helpful in outlining the basic deductions available to you. But you may also need to do some additional research if you have problems.

An all-purpose reference tool is the IRS's Publication 17, *Your Federal Income Tax.* It's quite comprehensive and, for the most part, is written in straightforward language. In the back of the 192-page book is a list of individual tax subjects discussed in the IRS's "500 series" of booklets. The booklets, which are excerpted and expanded from Publication 17, cover just about any topic a typical taxpayer might be interested in. They run a few pages each. All of these IRS publications are free; a call to your local IRS office is all it takes to get them.

There are drawbacks to IRS publications, however. First, they give only the IRS's view of the law and ignore court decisions that favor taxpayers. (For example, the IRS's treatment of office-in-home expenses. The IRS maintains you must compare the hours of actual use of the office to the hours of total availability and use a twenty-four-hour day as the basis for computation. But the Tax Court has held that allocations should be based on hours of normal use, *excluding* time spent working away from home or sleeping.) A second drawback is that these materials, prepared by the federal agency that is *the* authority on tax law, have no greater legal standing than any other self-help tax publication, and you cannot cite their advice as a defense if you are audited.

An alternative to the IRS books is one of the tax guides put out by commercial publishers. One generally regarded as excellent is J. K. Lasser's *Your Income Tax* (Simon and Schuster, $2.95), but you could well find one of the others more useful. To compare tax books, select a subject of particular pertinence to your situation alimony, perhaps. Then compare the treatment it gets in different publications. First, see if the subject is listed in the book's table of contents or index; if not, cross the book off your list. Then compare the length, depth, and clarity of the discussion of your topic. See if the book contains helpful examples of how to apply the law. See if it mentions court decisions that are contrary to the IRS's position. And see if it has a complete set of tax forms, as well as tables for computing your gasoline tax and state sales tax.

Some guidebooks are merely reprints of the IRS's Publication 17 with a different cover. These include Arco Publishing Co.'s version for $1.25 and DMR Publications' version for $1.95. Obviously, there's no reason to pay for information the government provides free.

Your local public library may provide you with information. Most library collections include publications on preparation of tax returns. Some libraries may also sponsor programs to help you with federal and state tax returns.

2. Help from the IRS

Although we have a tax system of "voluntary compliance," in which taxpayers are supposed to assess themselves, the IRS does accept some responsibility for helping taxpayers arrive at the correct figure. Through its Taxpayer Service Division, the IRS provides three basic types of assistance without charge:

1. **Telephone advice.** Toll-free telephone lines are available in all fifty-eight IRS districts. You can call for advice on tax computation problems as well as for help on such problems as tracing lost refund checks. During the filing season in 1975, the IRS got almost seventeen million calls. Those likely to get the most out of the telephone service are articulate taxpayers who know exactly what questions they want answered. You may run into problems if your questions are vague.

2. **Actual computation of your tax by mail.** The IRS will do your figuring for you if you use the short form, 1040A. The IRS will also help you with the long form, 1040, under two conditions: You must take the standard deduction, and you must have adjusted gross income (the income figure on line 15 of your form) of $20,000 or less derived *only* from wages, salary, tips, dividends, interest, pensions, and annuities. If you claim a retirement income credit (line 17 of the form), the IRS will also do that computation. The latter is not an offer to be taken lightly. One IRS official says: "People are so confused [about the retirement income credit] that they tend not to use it, and when they do use it, they make mistakes." The IRS will also compute the new earned income credit on the 1040A or 1040. To have the government figure out your tax, fill in the basic identification and income information on the form you use and mail it to the IRS by April 15.

3. Walk-in tax help. The IRS will prepare, or help you prepare, your return at one of its thousand or so offices. National policy is to limit complete preparation to persons who cannot do their own computations because of a disability (including illiteracy) : IRS policy is also to do tax preparation, workload permitting, for those who would otherwise be unwilling to fill out their own forms.

If you need only moral support and answers to a few questions, the IRS will assist you in filling out your return through its "self-help" program. In practice, this means that one IRS employe will help five or six taxpayers go through their returns, line by line. Taxpayers with dissimilar problems are often grouped together, without much privacy, so you may have to be patient (and thick-skinned) to get answers to your questions. In general, personalized one-to-one service is a luxury the IRS cannot afford to provide.

In 1975, the minimum educational requirements and training for employes in the division were upgraded. There are now two basic types of assisters: *taxpayer service representatives*, who must have two years of education beyond high school or the equivalent work experience; and *taxpayer service specialists*, who must have a college degree and accounting skills or the equivalent in experience. Taxpayer service representatives make up about 70 percent of the work force in the division. They receive an impressive amount of formal preseason training compared with preparers who work for commercial tax services: five weeks of classroom study and one week of simulation training. But many of them are still green. An IRS survey found that 37 percent of the taxpayer service representatives had been on the job only one year or less.

The IRS has also instituted a series of procedural improvements. It is testing its tax assisters to measure how well they have grasped the material they've been taught. It is encouraging novices to refer complicated tax questions to more knowledgeable employes. It is monitoring the advice given over the telephone. And it is reviewing the accuracy of returns prepared in its offices before they are sent out for final processing.

Now for the bad news. The impetus behind all the IRS's self-improvement measures is the error rate on advice given by its employes—it ranges from high to inexcusable.

The IRS makes its best showing with telephone inquiries. Various studies indicate the assisters give the wrong answer about 20 to 25 percent of the time. But the studies point up another drawback in calling the IRS for help: long delays. A 1974 study by the General Accounting Office reported that 36 percent of the calls received busy signals and 14 percent of the calls placed on hold were "lost." Another survey, conducted in 1975 by a House subcommittee, showed similar results. On one occasion, a call was placed on hold for 14½ minutes. When the person hung up and placed the call again, a recorded message announced the IRS office had closed for the day.

The IRS receives its lowest marks, however, on the returns its employes prepare or help to prepare. An internal survey conducted in 1975 by IRS agents posing as taxpayers showed that assisters handling relatively simple tax problems computed the wrong tax 72 percent of the time. About 18 percent of the returns contained mathematical errors and about 70 percent contained errors in applying the tax law. The cumulative dollar amount of the errors favored the government by a three-to-two ratio; that is, the government gained through error $3 in taxes for every $2 it gave up. The most frequent errors involved questions of casualty losses, moving expenses, and excess Social Security tax. In one case, an IRS employe added exemptions to income, instead of subtracting them, increasing the tax by almost $700.

A more comprehensive survey based on random audits of 1971 returns came up with similar results. The study compared the error rates of returns completed by various types of preparers, including the unassisted taxpayer, IRS Taxpayer Service, local tax services, national tax services, public accountants, and CPAs. (The IRS defined an error as a tax change of more than $1 after audit.) The study showed that, overall, IRS employes made mistakes 55 percent of the time. The error rate rose to about 74 percent, however, on returns with itemized deductions, and to an astounding 100 percent on returns with income from small corporations or partnerships.

Dismal as this record is, a preliminary report prepared for the Administrative Conference, an independent federal agency that spent a year studying the IRS, said: "Experienced observers believe that commercial, and perhaps professional, preparation is not as competent as IRS preparation." The complexities of the law can trip up even experienced tax lawyers.

IRS assistance has drawbacks other than uncertain accuracy. For one thing, IRS help is thinly spread. The IRS maintains about a thousand offices during tax season (a small number compared with H & R Block, which has blanketed the country with about seven times that many). Another problem is the lack of such basic equipment as calculators and adding machines.

You should know that you literally cannot depend on the advice the IRS gives you. In 1974, the U.S. Tax Court considered a case in which a taxpayer had suffered a $13,000 net operating loss on his business and followed IRS advice in claiming a loss-carryback adjustment. The IRS later reduced the adjustment. The case wound up in Tax

Court when the businessman complained about the reduction. The court commended him for seeking IRS help but said it's "well-settled" that erroneous IRS advice isn't binding.

The IRS does your federal return only, not your federal *and* state returns, as do commercial preparers. (But many states will help you do your state return for free. We contacted revenue offices in seven states—California, Illinois, Massachusetts, Michigan, New York, Ohio, and Pennsylvania—and each office said it gives taxpayers free assistance.)

If you visit the IRS, there are two additional points to keep in mind. Assisters are required to stamp and sign each return they prepare or help to prepare; some may be reluctant to do so. And some overzealous assisters may try to "audit" you on the spot by making you substantiate every deduction. But that's not their function, and it's against IRS rules. If you have a complaint on this score, first ask for a supervisor. If you're not satisfied, complain in writing to the Director of the Taxpayer Service Division and the Director of the Internal Audit Division, IRS, 1111 Constitution Avenue, Washington, D.C. 20224.

3. Help from a Local Tax Service

Until about twenty years ago, the IRS would prepare any tax return free. But the increasing number of taxpayers and complicated changes in the tax law forced it to limit this preparation service in the early 1950s to those who are unable or unwilling to do it themselves. Thus was born the commercial tax preparation industry.

At present, some 200,000 to 250,000 persons (no one knows the exact number) hold themselves up as tax consultants. There are no national standards, so virtually anyone who wants to can set up shop and hang out a sign.

Often, local tax service is provided by individuals who operate out of rented storefronts during the tax season and disappear after April 15.

The IRS believes tax preparation is a legitimate business, and Commissioner Donald C. Alexander has testified that it's not the IRS's job "to be avenging angels." Yet the IRS assumed that role a few years ago when it ordered a national crackdown on various return preparers, especially those it suspected of dishonesty. The campaign resulted in criminal action against more than one-third of the preparers examined. As a byproduct, some 250,000 tax returns that probably would have escaped scrutiny were audited simply because they were done by suspect preparers.

Although the IRS has discontinued this surveillance program on a national level, local offices still monitor some commercial preparers. Thus, if you innocently go to a dishonest local tax service, your chances of being audited may be greater than normal.

IRS statistics indicate a strong chance your return will be incorrectly prepared by a local tax service. Indeed, the study of 1971 returns referred to earlier showed that the error rate on returns done by local tax services was generally higher than that on returns done by other types of preparers. Usually, the wisest course is to avoid a local tax service, unless it has better credentials than simply a sign in the window (see page 55).

A brief word about the *computer tax services* that are beginning to appear on the scene. There's no magic in having a machine do computations. Tax preparation work is only as good as the questions that elicit the data that go into the computer. The actual computations should be done in addition to, but never as a substitute for, basic brain work.

4. Help from H & R Block, et al.

The picture is somewhat improved with the national tax services. The largest of these is H & R Block, which in 1975 prepared about 14 percent of all long forms filed (it did not prepare the short form until 1976). Many of our comments about this industry giant—which is almost thirty times larger than its closest competitor—apply to the other national tax services as well, most of which model their business methods on Block's.

Probably the primary reason for H & R Block's popularity is its convenience. During tax season it maintains some 7,200 offices and keeps them open nights and weekends. It employs about 43,000 preparers during the peak period.

Some of the company's growth is undoubtedly due to its promises, unique in the established tax preparation industry. One is its much publicized pledge to pay any interest and penalties assessed by the IRS if a client is forced to pay an extra tax as the result of a company error (neither Block nor any other preparer will pay the additional tax, however). The company is mum on the specific amount of interest and penalties it paid in 1975 but told CU the amount was so small it was handled out of petty cash. The latest public figures are for fiscal year 1972, when president Henry Bloch (he spells it with an "h") told Congress his firm paid out $139,159—a lot of money, but only a fraction of 1 percent of company volume.

Block also promises to accompany a taxpayer to the IRS office if the person is audited. (Note, however, that IRS rules *require* that a preparer appear as a witness and answer questions about how the return was prepared, if requested to appear by the IRS.) Block employs generally cannot represent taxpayers in adversary proceedings before the higher levels of the IRS, though; only CPAs, lawyers, and enrolled agents can do that.

Most Block customers are low- and moderate-income people (in 1974, 82 percent of its clients had incomes below $15,000), and the company's fees are tailored accordingly. The company charges $6 for the short form; the fee for the long form with Schedule A (itemized deductions) and Schedule B (interest and dividends) varies, depending on the complexity. In 1975, Block's average fee was about $17. Block also has an "executive service" for taxpayers with more complex returns; fees start at $25.

All fees include the preparation of state returns. But they are minimum charges and assume the taxpayer can provide the necessary information in an organized, systematic way. If your records are disorganized, you will probably pay more than the minimum.

Block applies the production-line technique to its operation. The general procedure is for a taxpayer to be taken on a first-come, first-served basis (no appointments, except for executive-service customers). The preparer interviews the client, does the basic computations, and then figures the tax. The return is then supposed to be checked for both procedural and mathematical accuracy. (Generally, new employes are expected to check one return for every return they prepare; the checking function is not reserved for experienced personnel, as in many CPA firms.) Five or six days later, the taxpayer can pick up the completed return at the Block office.

Block's stated policy is that anyone who works for the company must take a basic eighty-hour training course. There is no educational requirement; anyone who pays the $75 fee can enroll. To be hired, students must get a satisfactory appraisal from their instructor and handle a couple of brief quizzes in a "reasonable fashion." The company says it doesn't know how many students actually pass muster, but previous company statements indicate that 67 to 75 percent wind up as employes.

The lack of educational requirements and formal testing procedures points up a major problem with Block: the uneven quality of its preparers. Its employes are seasonal part-time workers who often are moonlighting; they have included salespeople, secretaries, construction workers, college students, and housewives. Some may be moonlighting accountants.

Block spot-checks the accuracy of work performed by its employes the same way the IRS does—by having other employes pose as taxpayers. But the error rate is kept private. "The figures are not combined in a meaningful way that would be of use to you," CU was told, "but if an office has a problem, we sweep in and fix it." Judging from IRS statistics, Block isn't using the broom often enough.

The statistics are from a study, referred to earlier, that examined a sample of 1971 returns prepared by various types of preparers, including national tax services. The "national tax service" category didn't name names. But Block commands the lion's share of that market. (Of 8,770,000 returns prepared in 1975 by national tax services, Block prepared 8,235,000 returns, or about 94 percent.) The IRS survey showed that on low-income returns with itemized deductions—the type of returns in which Block specializes—the error rate was 82 percent. This was a higher error rate than on returns prepared with IRS help, or by public accountants and CPAs. On returns with income from partnerships or small corporations, national tax services did even worse, making mistakes 87 percent of the time. Public accountants and CPAs made significantly fewer errors than that.

A study conducted by the General Accounting Office (GAO) and released in 1976 gave somewhat similar results. Like the IRS study, the GAO report was based on randomly selected returns but used a different measure of error than the IRS had. The GAO compared the "percent of tax change"—the amount of the error after audit, divided by the amount of the tax originally paid. In the complex tax area of professional and business income (computed on Schedule C), commercial preparers had a percent tax change of 82 percent while professionals had a percent tax change of 60 percent.

This last statistic points up a major problem in going to H & R Block: Many of its employes are not equipped to deal with complicated returns and may not even recognize a complex situation when faced with one. Two adverse court decisions speak to this point.

In 1973, the Nevada Supreme Court ordered a Block franchise-holder to pay $100,000 in punitive and actual damages to former clients because of mistakes made in preparing their partnership returns. The returns were prepared by a former construction worker who, according to the court, "had received no formal training." The court said the evidence showed "willful and wanton misrepresentation" in Block's advertising and internal business practices, "specifically aimed at deceiving the members of the public who might rely on [the company] for tax expertise."

The court said Block made "no effort to hire employes with even rudimentary skill in accounting or in the preparation of tax returns." And it noted that Block's internal manual instructs its office managers to "counter inquiries concerning the qualifications of employes by saying that '[the company] has been preparing taxes for 20 years.'"

A similar credibility gap between Block's public assertions and its private policies came to light in the trial of a Block franchise-holder in Maryland. The mistake involved an improper business loss on a return prepared by someone new to the job. When the Block franchise-holder, a former baker with an eleventh-grade education, refused to pay interest and penalties on the additional tax assessed—as company advertising promises—the clients filed suit. The state appeals court said both the preparer and the franchise-holder "lacked the training, experience or competence to understand the requirements of the business tax returns which they prepared." The franchise-holder was ultimately ordered to pay the clients about $670 in damages.

One reason for the company's inept handling of business returns probably lies in its training tools. The three basic reference materials are the IRS's Publication 17, the company's simplified version of basic tax law, and a commercial guide to tax law for nonprofessionals. The use of other, less superficial sources, such as collections of tax court decisions frequently consulted by CPAs when dealing with difficult tax subjects, isn't standard operating procedure in many Block offices.

Given the uneven quality of Block tax preparation, you should entrust it with only the simplest, most routine type of return. Even then, you're not safe. The New York City Department of Consumer Affairs received a letter from a former Block client in 1975 who complained that the company's preparer hadn't even correctly computed her income, listed on two sets of W-2 forms. The obvious mistake had escaped Block's checking system as well. The office manager's response was to recompute the tax and offer the client "gift certificates" for the following year's preparation (company policy prohibits refunds of fees and calls for the distribution of gift certificates instead).

Another drawback is that Block's wage structure encourages workers to compensate for low basic pay by high volume of commission fees. Block pays its new employes the minimum wage ($2.30 an hour) as a draw against 20 percent commission on the fees for returns they prepare. The more returns a preparer completes, the more the person earns. Thus a conscientious worker who lavishes time on each return does not earn as much as a high-volume operator. Result: a revolving-door approach to clients.

A look inside Block's operations is revealing. A CPA who worked for Block's main Manhattan office in 1971 testified before Congress that the office manager was an undergraduate student, and his fellow tax preparers included a toy salesman and an unemployed stockbroker. The checking system was superficial at best. A student hired to do that specific job was expected to check thirty-five to forty returns an hour. And when the CPA was assigned to checking duties, he found errors 50 to 60 percent of the time—and more than once was ordered to "take it easy." As things got hectic just before April 15, the CPA testified, the checking function was abandoned entirely.

As we noted earlier, Block's operating procedures have been copied by its competitors. It would be prudent to assume, therefore, that they share both the general strengths and weaknesses of the industry giant. Chief competitors are:

Tax Corporation of America. This firm, the second largest in terms of volume, did 300,000 returns in 1975. It has offices in thirty-eight states but is concentrated mainly in the West. Applicants go through a preliminary screening before they are admitted to the company's sixty-hour training course; trainees automatically become employes on completion of the course. They are paid on commission. Tax Corp.'s procedure in preparing returns varies somewhat from Block's. Employes interview clients in the clients' homes and do a preliminary tax computation there. Then they feed the information into a computer, which does the actual mathematics. The basic charge is $25 for an itemized long form with schedules A and B, and $5 to $8 for a short form. The company pays interest and penalties on both mathematical and procedural errors and will accompany clients on an audit. Consumers Union has received one letter complaining about the company. A Maryland woman said she had grossly overpaid her tax in the two years she relied on the company. She eventually received a $1,570 refund from the IRS.

Beneficial's Income Tax Service. A unit of the giant consumer loan company, Beneficial Corp., it is the next largest national tax service and prepared 125,000 returns in 1975. Beneficial provides tax help from 1,350 of the finance company's loan offices around the country. It trains its workers for sixty hours and also hires some former Block employes. They are paid salary and commission. It charges $6.50 for the short form and $14 for a long form with schedules A and B. It will pay interest and penalties on mathematical errors only and doesn't promise to accompany you on an audit.

Potential clients of Beneficial should be aware of a legal action regarding its customer practices (still unresolved as of this writing). The Federal Trade Commission is trying to prevent the company from using the term "Instant Tax Refund"—in fact, just a normal consumer loan, with interest charges—and from using confidential tax information to solicit loan customers. (The company says its ads mention that the "Instant Refund" is a loan, and that customers who are solicited for loans sign consent forms.) Until legal action is completed, Beneficial is free to continue these practices.

Mr. Tax of America. The fourth largest of the national tax services, the company did 110,000 returns in 1975. It operates in twenty-five states, mainly in the Midwest and

Southwest. Its employes are trained for seventy to eighty hours and are paid salary plus commission. The company's charge is about $20 for a long form with schedules A and B, and $10 for a nonitemized long form. It pays penalties on both procedural and mathematical errors and will accompany a taxpayer on an audit.

How to Deal with a Commercial Preparer. The initials "CPA" are the only badge of competence among commercial tax preparers. But few taxpayers require a CPA's skills and the high attendant fees. Other commercial preparers can do a good job with routine tax returns; a lot depends on their training, experience, and procedures. Here are some facts you should find out about any commercial preparer who is not a CPA.

1. Does the preparer have at least two years of college? A college degree with some accounting courses is preferable.

2. Has the preparer passed a formal tax training course? The IRS gives its employes 190 hours or so of training, and national tax services provide 60 to 80 hours. Don't assume that just because someone works for a large tax service, the person has taken the company's training course. That's not always the case.

3. How long has the individual been preparing returns? Two years' experience should be the minimum.

4. Is the preparer in business year round? Avoid places that close up shop after April 15. If you're audited, you want access to the person who prepared your returns or to the office that employed the person and has copies of your records.

5. Does the preparer sign the return? The IRS requires this, so insist on it. This fixes some of the responsibility for the accuracy of the return on the preparer. But you are the

one who is basically responsible, and you are the one who must pay any additional tax the IRS may eventually decide is due.

6. Does the preparer keep copies of the return for at least three years? That's how long the statute of limitations runs on most returns. Be sure you get a copy of your return (with the preparer's name and address on it) and keep the copy in your files for at least three years.

7. Does the preparer try different ways of figuring your tax? Using the standard deductions or tax tables may be all that's required for simple returns. But other methods, such as income averaging, may be called for in special situations—say, if family income has jumped because a wife has returned to work.

Beware of a preparer who guarantees you a refund or who suggests you have the refund sent to his or her office. (If you have a refund coming, but plan to move after filing your return, be sure to note your new address on the return.) Never sign a blank return—it's like signing a blank check. And never sign a return that's been filled out in pencil because the computations can later be changed without your knowledge.

Check over the return before you mail it. Some unscrupulous preparers have been known to create phantom dependents and phony charitable deductions in order to arrive at a refund. At the very least, be sure the number of personal exemptions is correct and that the income listed on the return matches your W-2 forms and other documents.

Get an estimate of the cost of preparation beforehand, and find out if it covers both federal and state returns (local ones, too, if needed). Get a receipt after you've paid; the fee is tax-deductible next year. If the preparer ties the fee to the amount of the refund claimed, it would be wise to look elsewhere.

5. Help from an Enrolled Agent

A step up from the typical storefront preparer, national or local, is one of the fifteen thousand or so enrolled agents—preparers who have passed a stiff Treasury Department examination. In addition to preparing your return, enrolled agents can argue points of tax law on your behalf, negotiate settlements, and take your case through the appeals levels within the IRS.

The nine-hour examination they take covers tax accounting for individuals, partnerships, corporations, trusts, and estates. Only 60 percent pass, so certification offers some indication of proficiency.

There are no educational standards, and some recent enrolled agents have included a sheet metal contractor and an off-duty airline pilot. The IRS is rather hazy about what kind of person becomes an enrolled agent. Other sources estimate that one-tenth are former IRS tax auditors (who don't need to take the examination to be enrolled) and one-third are public accountants. Such additional experience and background might inspire increased confidence in the training of an enrolled agent.

There may be some real problems in locating enrolled agents. Only eight states have five hundred or more enrolled agents: California, Florida, Illinois, Michigan, New York, Ohio, Pennsylvania, and Texas. If you don't live in one of those states, your chances of finding an enrolled agent are slim.

Even if you live in one of the eight states, you may have trouble finding the names of agents in your area. That's because the IRS, having ascertained that these people are knowledgeable enough to pass the government test on tax law, refuses to allow them to advertise this fact to the public, not even by a listing in the Yellow Pages.

At the time that CU first prepared this report, the IRS claimed you could get a list of enrolled agents in your area by writing to the district director of the nearest IRS office (the charge, if any, set by the local office). But don't hold your breath waiting. On the advice of the IRS's national office in Washington, a CU staff member wrote to the director of the New York City district office in November and again in December 1975. She finally received an acknowledgment in January directing her back to IRS Washington headquarters. But the list did not arrive until July. The IRS now says that it will furnish the names of enrolled agents in your state for a small charge (the fee depends on the number of pages the state listing covers). Address your request to Chief, Disclosure Staff, Internal Revenue Service, Ben Franklin Station, Washington, D.C. 20044.

A California trade group, the Association of Enrolled Agents, said it would provide the names of the three enrolled agents closest to your home if you send a stamped, self-addressed envelope to the association at 8155 Van Nuys Boulevard, Suite 1114, Panorama City, Calif. 91402.

6. Help from a Public Accountant

One dictionary defines an accountant as a "person whose profession is inspecting and auditing personal and commercial accounts." There are two basic types of public accountants: those who are certified and those who aren't.

Accountants in the latter group are in accounting by virtue of aptitude, training, or happenstance. Only sixteen states have any licensing requirements at all, and their standards vary widely.* Elsewhere in the country, anyone

*The sixteen states with licensing requirements for public accountants are: Alabama, Alaska, Arizona, Georgia, Indiana, Iowa, Montana, New Hampshire, New Mexico, Ohio, Oklahoma, Oregon, South Carolina, South Dakota, Tennessee, and Vermont.

who wants to can set up shop as a public accountant. There are no minimum educational requirements and no tests an applicant must pass. Some may have studied accounting in college, but others may have never even taken a high school course in bookkeeping. The National Society of Public Accountants considers "anyone who is in the public practice of accountancy" a public accountant.

The only requirement of the organization, which represents not quite 30 percent of the fifty-five thousand or so public accountants in the country, is that a member observe its code of ethics (it forbids advertising, among other things). The organization also sponsors a continuing education program that can serve as a yardstick for gauging an individual's professional interest in keeping current. The trade group estimates that about one-third of its members have also passed the IRS examination and are enrolled agents who can represent clients before the IRS. (You can get a list of society members by writing to the National Society of Public Accountants, 1717 Pennsylvania Avenue N.W., Washington, D.C. 20006.)

Public accountants generally cater to small businesses or individuals of moderate means. Most of their clients earn between $5,000 and $20,000. A 1971 survey by the national society indicated they prepared about seven million individual returns—almost the same number that H & R Block prepared that year. They charge a little more than national tax services, but less than CPAs. In 1975, their average charge for an itemized long form was $39; regional averages ranged from a low of $32 in the Northwest to a high of $48 in the Far West.

The IRS error-rate study indicates that public accountants make a respectable showing compared with local and national tax services, but don't measure up as well when compared with CPAs and the IRS.

A well-qualified public accountant could be a good compromise choice if your return is too complicated for a national tax service but not complicated enough to justify the expense of a CPA. Because the entry requirements of the profession are so vague, it's not enough just to consult the Yellow Pages. If you live in one of the sixteen states with licensing laws, ask if the person has met state requirements. Then find out if the person is a member of the national society and has been accredited under the society's continuing education program. Finally, ask if the person is an enrolled agent. The more of these hurdles a public accountant has jumped, the more dependable the help is likely to be.

7. Help from a CPA

CPAs are the top of the line in tax help. They generally must be college graduates or have equivalent work experience. They must also pass a tough two-and-a-half-day examination—and only 10 percent do the first time around. To take the examination, they must first have worked under the supervision of a CPA (the amount of working experience required varies from state to state). There are roughly 160,000 or so CPAs in the country; they generally specialize in corporate accounting and auditing, not individual tax-return preparation. You can expect them to prepare fairly accurate returns, no matter how complex the subject: IRS statistics indicate their error rate is consistently lower than that of all other types of paid tax-preparers.

You probably should visit a CPA if you have a complicated economic life. You can consider yours a "complicated" economic life if your income figure is higher than $30,000 and includes income from tax-exempt securities, investment property, royalties, a trust fund, or hobbies. Yours is also a "complicated" economic life if you bought or sold a house or condominium; bought or sold securities; suffered a casualty loss; had deductible expenses for dependents other than your immediate family; used personal assets, such as your car or house, partly for business; gave gifts valued at $3,000 or more; or worked abroad.

You might also benefit from a CPA's advice if there is a major change in your lifestyle due to marriage, divorce, death in the family, or retirement; these all may have tax consequences, as may a large increase in a family's income, which sometimes occurs when a wife returns to work.

CPAs are automatically authorized to represent clients before the IRS. But you should be sure the CPA will do so in case you are audited; and find out what the approximate charge will be. Another service CPAs can provide is tax planning—help in arranging your financial affairs to minimize your taxes. They can do this, for example, by suggesting the formation of trusts, recommending certain types of investment property or the sale of certain securities.

CPAs tend to charge the highest fees of all preparers. Generally, the minimum charge is $50 for a very simple return. A somewhat more complicated return will run at least $150 to $200. And the fee could go as high as $500 to $600 if the session includes tax planning. If you're on a tight budget, you might visit a CPA once to see how the accountant sets up your return, and use it as a guide in following years—until there's a major change in tax law or your financial circumstances.

The best way to find a CPA is to ask around among friends or colleagues whose work is similar to your own. If you're an architect, for example, a CPA who has handled other architects' returns will probably be aware of your special tax problems. You can also ask for recommendations from your employer or from the tax department of a large CPA firm. Be sure to mention who recommended you.

It may ensure careful work on your return, for the CPA should realize that a sloppy job will mean the loss of more than just one client. Look for small firms or an individual practitioner. Big CPA firms generally restrict their practices to large corporations and the executives who run them. Find out who will actually be preparing your work and what supervision, if any, the person receives. In many top CPA firms, junior personnel do the computations, but their work is checked by the senior CPAs on staff. Ask if the CPA keeps copies of returns for at least three years, and obtain a copy for yourself to keep in *your* files for at least three years.

Lawyers also handle tax matters, but they tend to provide advice rather than preparation. If you use a lawyer, choose one who took accounting in law school and who is experienced in preparing tax returns. Except in small towns, the number of returns they prepare is relatively small, usually for clients in high tax brackets. It's not uncommon, however, for lawyers to review returns prepared by CPAs.

Storefront Accountants for the Poor. Dedicated young CPAs in a handful of cities are providing free top-notch tax help for the "working poor." Operating out of storefronts donated by community groups, they serve families with incomes of up to $10,000.

The largest of these groups is Community Tax Aid in New York City. A nonprofit organization with a minuscule budget, it has prepared nearly thirty thousand returns since it was founded in 1969. Eligibility for Community Tax Aid is based on a sliding scale of family size and income.

Similar CPA volunteer organizations are located in Los Angeles, Denver, Minneapolis, Philadelphia, Newark, N.J., Charlotte, N.C., and Hartford, Conn. For more information on these programs, or if you're a CPA or lawyer and want help in starting your own community tax service, contact Community Tax Aid, Box 1040, Cathedral Station, New York, N.Y. 10025.

Not all volunteer programs are run by CPAs. For example, the tax accounting faculty at California State University in Hayward sponsors Volunteer Income Tax Assistance, which offers free help to the "working poor" in the area.

Recommendations

Tax preparation is at best an imperfect art. No matter who does your return, there's a chance that a hard-nosed IRS auditor will interpret the law differently from the person who filled out your form.

Unfortunately, the complicated tax code remains the basic obstacle to preparing accurate tax returns. Congress has virtually legislated the commercial tax preparation industry into existence without controlling it. Although reforms for regulating tax preparers were introduced in Congress as long as twenty years ago, none have become law. Just a few locales—California, Idaho, Oregon, and New York City—have laws governing the conduct of tax preparers. Those most qualified to help taxpayers—CPAs, public accountants, and enrolled agents—are not permitted to advertise to the public, while those least qualified have almost free rein to make advertising claims.

Here is CU's advice for preparing your tax in this imperfect world.

1. If you have confidence in yourself, if you like the scholarship involved in looking things up, if you have the time to spare, if you have a calculator or a good head for figures, and if you lead a simple economic life, do it yourself.

2. If you lead a simple economic life, but really don't want

to do it yourself, visit an IRS office for help. The IRS makes errors, true, but only a CPA is likely to do a lot better.

3. In general, stay away from local, temporary storefront preparers (though not all are unreliable). Try a national tax service only if your return is routine, and if you're willing to pay something for service more personal than that dispensed by the IRS. Never go to a national tax service with a business return or a complicated personal situation unless you're confident that the personnel in the office are unusually well qualified.

4. If your return is somewhat more than routine, visit an enrolled agent or a public accountant.

5. If your financial life is filled with knotty complexities, see a CPA or a lawyer.

WHEN THE IRS COMES CALLING

Two-thirds of the roughly two million taxpayers whose returns are audited in 1977 will be told they owe Uncle Sam money. That's an intimidating statistic for ordinary taxpayers who may disagree with the findings, particularly for those who can't afford professional representation. The staff of the Administrative Conference, an independent government agency that spent a year investigating the IRS, has found that unrepresented taxpayers who try to protest are "simply overmatched." The staff recommended that Congress establish a "taxpayer assistance center" where citizens who dispute IRS audit findings could get independent legal advice. Nothing has come of that idea, but persistent taxpayers with the time and resources to contest an audit will generally find the battle worthwhile. Taxpayers who appeal audit results will, on average, pay less than half of what they would have paid had they allowed the IRS findings to stand. So it makes sense to know how a tax audit comes about—and how to deal with it.

The audit process begins at one of ten IRS service centers around the country. There, computers and IRS clerks routinely check for such obvious errors as missing signatures, missing Social Security numbers, and mathematical mistakes. A magnetic tape with the pertinent information from each return then goes to the National Computer Center in Martinsburg, W.Va., where each return is rated by computer for its "error potential."

There are a number of different formulas for figuring a return's error potential, but just how they work is one of Washington's best kept secrets. Variables probably include such things as the amount of income and its source, the number and types of dependents, the size and nature of certain itemized deductions, and marital status.

When the computer kicks out a return with a high score —that is, a return with a high potential for error—a human being called a classifying officer inspects it to see if there's an obvious, or innocent, explanation for the score. It therefore makes sense to attach substantiation for unusual or large deductions when making out a tax return. Someone with large medical expenses, for instance, may head off an audit by attaching a note explaining the nature of the illness and copies of hospital or doctors' bills. (Never attach originals—they could be lost.)

If the classifying officer sees no ready explanation for the return's high score, the questionable return is forwarded to the IRS audit division for follow-up.

About three-fourths of all returns that are audited were originally selected by the computer. The others are manually selected under various IRS programs designed to find specific types of tax problems. High-income taxpayers (probably those with incomes well over $100,000 a year) can expect an automatic audit. So can persons who were assessed extra tax after a state audit. (Since the IRS and the states routinely exchange tax information, someone audited by the federal government can expect a state audit to follow as well.) If the IRS audits a taxpayer's return and finds an error, it may review that taxpayer's return the following year just to see if the error is repeated.

Divorced persons stand a good chance of an audit if the IRS has questions about alimony or dependency deductions. Taxpayers who go to commercial preparers whom the IRS is investigating for fraud may find their returns under scrutiny, too. The IRS also relies on informants, who receive rewards ranging from 1 to 10 percent of the money collected as a result of their tips.

Because the IRS has found that the tax compliance habits of citizens vary by income level, it audits a different percentage of returns in different income brackets. If your adjusted gross income last year was under $10,000, your chances of an audit are one in fifty-five; if it was between $10,000 and $50,000, your chances are one in forty; and if it was over $50,000, your chances are one in eight.

There are five major types of IRS audits for ordinary taxpayers. All are basically routine checks to see that the taxpayers can substantiate certain items on their returns.

The simplest audit, under the so-called *unallowables program*, is conducted back at step one, the service center. The service center reviews returns for items that are obviously not in accordance with the law. The error found most frequently is that people take more than the standard deduction. Other frequent errors include incorrect claims of head-of-household status, claims of charitable contributions to organizations that did not qualify for charitable status, and deductions of more than the permitted limit of

$400 a month for child-care expenses.

Taxpayers audited under this program receive a computer-printed notice proposing a "correction" in the tax. The IRS rarely makes a mistake in correcting "unallowable" entries. But taxpayers should check out the government's explanation for the change, as well as its arithmetic. If there's any question about the change, or if there's no explanation for the "correction," taxpayers have the same right to protest as they do with any other type of audit.

The second type of audit, a *correspondence audit*, is, as its name implies, a letter from the IRS questioning a single tax issue, such as medical deductions. The letter will indicate what item on the return is being questioned and will ask the taxpayer to mail copies of supporting documents to the IRS. Substantiation might be in the form of a receipt or a canceled check, or it might be merely a written explanation of how the person arrived at a particular figure entered on the return. In a correspondence audit, the IRS waits for you to send some kind of substantiation before proposing any changes in the tax bill.

An *office audit*, in which the taxpayer is asked to visit an IRS office to discuss the return, is what usually comes to mind when audits are mentioned. In fact, the vast majority of audits of individual tax returns are conducted this way. Typical issues explored at these audits include dependency exemptions, travel and entertainment expenses, income from tips, capital gains entries, and bad debts. The IRS notifies taxpayers of an office audit by a letter that states specifically the items to be covered at the interview. The interview usually lasts an hour or two.

The complex financial affairs of wealthy taxpayers, professional persons such as doctors and lawyers, and large corporations are usually handled through *field audits*. In a field audit, an IRS officer visits the taxpayer's home or office to inspect records that are usually too voluminous to move.

There are also *research audits*—audits of returns chosen at random from a scientific sample based on the ending digits of taxpayers' Social Security numbers. These audits represent less than 2 percent of all returns audited. But because they are selected as part of a research program to check how well taxpayers are complying with the law and to update the computer programs that select most returns for audit, the unlucky citizens audited at random are in for a much harder time than those selected for audit by other methods. In a research audit, the IRS requires taxpayers to substantiate every piece of information on their returns, right down to the last miscellaneous itemized deduction.

Office and correspondence audits are conducted by IRS employes known as office auditors, and field audits are conducted by employes called revenue agents. Taxpayers contacted by office auditors or revenue agents can rest assured their audits are probably routine. But taxpayers contacted by IRS employes who identify themselves as "special agents" should consult a lawyer. Special agents, who work for the Internal Revenue Service's intelligence division, are called in only on cases of suspected fraud, which is a criminal offense.

Notice of an audit, even an office audit, doesn't usually imply that you are suspected of criminal tax evasion. But the IRS wouldn't want to talk with you if it didn't think something was amiss with your return. You may well disagree with that assessment, and you have the right to assistance in voicing your disagreement to the IRS tax examiner.

If you are called in for an audit, you may bring a relative or friend for moral support (one person is usually the limit, however). You also have the right to be represented (in your absence, if you wish) by a lawyer, a CPA, or an "enrolled agent"—a person who has passed an IRS examination on tax law. The representative of a commercial preparer, such as H & R Block, can accompany you, but usually only to answer questions about how your return was prepared, not to argue your case.

Should the audit date chosen by the IRS be inconvenient, you have the right to reschedule the examination. (Ask for the first appointment of the day—the IRS tends to fall behind as the day progresses.) If you wind up with an auditor you consider unreasonable in interpreting the law, or if you have a personality conflict with an examiner, you can ask the auditor's supervisor to assign your case to someone else.

If the IRS serves you with a summons, you may decide to turn over records that will substantiate your return, even though personal papers are generally privileged. You are not required to turn over records that may be incriminating, although refusal to do so may make the auditor suspicious. The wisest course is to provide only those records directly related to the issue or issues in question. If the examiner wants a number of records to peruse at leisure, ask for a written list of precisely which records are needed.

An audit is basically an adversary proceeding. But unlike a court trial, where the defendant is presumed innocent until proved guilty, an audit places the burden of proof on the taxpayer. Therefore, a persuasive defense is important. Although a typical taxpayer probably doesn't need a lawyer's high-priced services to substantiate figures on the return, you should prepare for an audit in much the same way a lawyer prepares for a courtroom appearance. Marshal all the evidence you can get.

Third-party evidence can be particularly helpful in substantiating a questionable deduction. Let's assume a taxpayer is trying to justify a claimed casualty loss resulting from storm damage to a home. Photographs showing the condition of the house before and after the storm would help. So would a copy of a professional estimator's report on the cost of repair, and records indicating how much of the loss, if any, was reimbursed by insurance. If the loss was due to theft, a copy of a police report would indicate the incident was *bona fide* and reported to authorities. Taxpayers who are questioned about work-related travel and entertainment expenses will probably be asked to provide a letter from their employers stating whether or not the expenses were reimbursed and, if so, to what extent. Gather these records before the audit; many audits are held up because taxpayers fail to bring the proper records to the initial interview.

Income tax authorities advise most taxpayers to retain certain records, such as receipts for charitable contributions and medical expenses, for at least three years after the due date of the return.* The statute of limitations for auditing individual returns runs for three years, although the IRS tries to audit returns within twenty-six months of their filing deadline. Thus, returns due in April 1976 will remain in the audit hopper until June 1978. (The statute of limitations can be extended to six years, however, if taxpayers fail to report more than 25 percent of their income; and it can run indefinitely in cases of fraud.)

You should know something about the ground rules established by the IRS for an office audit. Agents who interview taxpayers in their offices are supplied with examination checksheets that list the items to be discussed. Auditors

*If you own a house, invest in the stock market, or collect paintings, stamps, coins, or the like, you should keep records on these holdings for as long as you own the property. When you sell these assets, your records will help to determine how much of the income you realize will be taxed.

are not permitted to expand the scope of the examination beyond the items on the checksheet—unless they find "an issue of significance" that was not noted on the sheet. But the taxpayer is under no obligation to answer questions about issues brought up for the first time at the audit. It's perfectly acceptable to tell the agent that you are not prepared to discuss the new subjects but that you will be glad to comply—by mail—once you have looked over your records in private.

Nor should you volunteer new information at the interview. Limit your answers to the subject or subjects that triggered the examination: those listed on the letter notifying you of the audit. (A lawyer recently audited because of high medical expenses wound up paying $58 in extra taxes because he showed his previous year's return to the auditor. After examining the return closely, the auditor discovered that the lawyer hadn't reported his local income-tax refund as income in the following year.)

Taxpayers are entitled to argue new points in their favor. If between the time you filed your return and the time of an audit you learn about significant deductions you might have taken, by all means mention them. Refunds were received by 5 percent of those audited in 1974.

When the examination is completed, the auditor will tell you what the results are. IRS studies on the results of office audits in fiscal year 1975 indicate that 24 percent of audited taxpayers with adjusted gross incomes between $10,000 and $50,000 were able to show that their returns were correct. Taxpayers in that income group who were assessed additional taxes owed an average of $230 each, including penalties.

An auditor's finding is merely a recommendation, not a final ruling. You can appeal to have it reversed or reduced. Keep that in mind if an auditor presses you to agree to an additional tax payment on the spot (examiners are under pressure to close a certain number of cases a day). Should you disagree with the recommendation, tell the auditor you want to think about it for a day or two. In that time, you might want to seek professional advice. Should you accept the auditor's finding, you'll be asked to sign a waiver agreement, known as Form 870. By signing this document, you agree to pay the extra tax, and you waive your rights to contest the finding in Tax Court. (You can later sue for a refund in United States District Court or the Court of Claims, but usually only wealthy taxpayers follow that course.)

Should you disagree with the examiner's recommendation, there are a number of options open. You can ask for an immediate meeting with the examiner's supervisor. If you fail to reach an agreement at this point, you can go through the formal appeals process discussed below.

If you believe you have been unfairly treated or harassed by your auditor, first complain to your auditor's supervisor. Should you get no satisfaction, write a letter to the chief of audit of your local IRS district office and send a copy to the IRS's inspection division at 1111 Constitution Avenue N.W., Washington, D.C. 20224.

How to Appeal an Audit

There is one basic appeals route with three major stops along the way. You can contest the finding through a conference at the IRS *district* level, where your audit was conducted. You can argue your case at a conference at the IRS *appellate* level, where it will be considered by the staff of one of the seven IRS regional offices. Or you can take your case to *court*, which is completely outside the IRS hierarchy. You don't have to appeal one step at a time. You can bypass the district conference and go straight to the appellate staff, or you can bypass both of these conferences and go straight to court.

Perhaps because auditors' findings are reviewed on appeal by more experienced IRS employes, or perhaps because taxpayers don't go to the trouble and expense of appealing unless they have a good case, those who do appeal often succeed in reducing the amount of additional tax recommended by the examiner. In appellate-level settlements during fiscal 1975, for instance, the IRS collected only 78 cents on the dollar from persons who appealed an extra assessment of $1,000 or less, 66 cents on the dollar from persons assessed between $1,000 and $10,000, and 57 cents on the dollar from taxpayers who appealed an extra assessment of between $10,000 and $50,000.

Nevertheless, the cost of an appeal often exceeds the potential gain for many small taxpayers, and 99 percent of them settle right after audit. Professional help is expensive. You can expect to pay a CPA or an attorney a fee of $25 an hour and up. In some instances, particularly when there's a large sum of money in dispute, they work on a contingency basis—that is, they base the fee on a fixed percentage of the money they may save you through appealing. Even when you argue your own case in the small case session of Tax Court, preparing for it may be time-consuming and may require you to take a day or two off from work.

If you do decide to protest, you should know that the IRS will do everything it can to convince you to settle as early as possible. It will urge you to resolve the matter through a conference at the district level, with an IRS mediator called a *district conferee*. To prevent "small" tax cases (those with a disputed tax of $2,500 or less) from going up the appeals ladder and clogging the courts, the IRS has given district conferees special flexibility in dealing with these cases.

One way the IRS allows conferees to settle small cases is by "splitting" issues. Say the IRS disputes the claim of a divorced father that a child of the marriage is his dependent rather than the mother's. Ordinarily, this is an all-or-nothing question, since only one parent can claim the child as a dependent. However, the conferee can settle the case by allowing the former husband to pay less than the entire amount of tax in dispute.

District conferees can base a settlement on their judgment of a taxpayer's chance of winning in court. If the chance is believed to be fifty-fifty, the conferee can offer to settle for half the disputed tax. The conferee can also settle a case by "trading" issues—conceding disputed medical deductions, say, in return for the taxpayer giving in on another item, perhaps disputed charitable deductions.

If you can't reach a settlement with the district conferee despite these special procedures, you can take your case to the next level of the IRS, the appellate division. Your case will be bumped up to an *appellate conferee* (usually someone with more legal background than a district conferee).

But in almost all cases, ordinary taxpayers who dispute an auditor's finding are probably best off taking their appeal directly to Tax Court, which is completely independent of the IRS. The court has two sessions: a regular session for large cases and a small case session for persons with $1,500 or less in dispute (more than 80 percent of those audited in 1975 fell into the latter category). The small case session is one place where the unrepresented taxpayer can get a sympathetic but impartial hearing quickly and inexpensively. You can argue your own case without a lawyer for just a $10 filing fee.

To bring your case before the court, you must ask the IRS to issue you a "statutory notice of deficiency," sometimes known as a "ninety-day letter," after the audit. This notice gives you ninety days to petition the court for a hearing. It's important that you file the petition (you should use certified mail) within ninety days of the date the IRS sends the notice; as many as 10 percent of the petitions the court receives are rejected because they are filed too late. Tax Court judges ride a "traveling circuit" to more than a hundred cities around the country. After the court receives the petition, it will assign your case to the city on the circuit that is closest to your home and will schedule your case for the next session in that city.

The small case session maintains an informal courtroom atmosphere. Taxpayers often present their cases while sitting at a table, with the personal records spread out before them. Hearsay evidence (second-hand evidence) is usually accepted. So are copies of documents, rather than originals. Affidavits are often acceptable substitutes for courtroom appearances of witnesses for the taxpayer.

The small case procedure has two drawbacks, however. First, there is no appeal; the decision of the judge is final. Second, there is no precedent, which means that even if one judge has previously considered a tax issue similar to your own and has ruled in favor of the taxpayer, that decision is not binding on the judge who considers your case.

If you feel shy about taking the IRS to court, consider this: In fiscal 1975, the Tax Court received 3,203 petitions to hear small tax cases. Nearly 80 percent of those were settled, most of them in last-minute negotiations between the taxpayer and the IRS. In those settlements, the IRS agreed to accept, on average, only 54 percent of the taxes it originally claimed were due. Of the small number of cases that actually came to trial, only 11 percent were decided in favor of the taxpayer. The IRS won 62 percent of the cases, and 27 percent were split decisions (decided partly in favor of the taxpayer and partly in favor of the government).

Since the IRS tries so hard to keep small cases out of court, it's likely that many taxpayers who won't agree to settle before trial are arguing hopeless cases based on what they think the law should be, rather than what it is. But there's nothing wrong in that. Congress created the small case procedure to give taxpayers a fresh forum in which to air their disputes with the IRS. For many of them, the satisfaction comes not from winning a fine point of tax law but in exercising their right to their day in court.

IRS Audit Guides

At tax time, financial magazines and business pages of newspapers are full of advertisements for books billed as *The Official IRS Audit Guide*. These books, which are priced at $5 or more, promise to divulge the IRS's trade secrets. But they're really just reprints of carefully edited sections of the *Internal Revenue Manual*. The same information is available from the IRS at a fraction of the cost.

There are six different IRS audit guides, but they tend to repeat the same information. The audit guides are primarily common-sense applications of the income tax laws and regulations explained in *Your Federal Income Tax* (IRS Publication 17), the all-purpose tax guide for individuals. Although audit guides do provide some clues to the direction an audit might take, the clues won't help a taxpayer prepare for a visit to the IRS. If everything on your return is legal, and if you can substantiate it, then you don't need a guide at all. If you've taken an improper deduction, the guides will only alert you to the fact that an examiner is likely to take a certain line of questioning designed to uncover your error.

There are no magic numbers indicating what the acceptable medical or charitable deductions are for your income bracket. Nor are there any hints to whether there is any deduction so small the IRS won't bother to check it.

If you are determined to order one of these guides, and if you have a simple nonbusiness return, the most helpful publication is *Tax Audit Guidelines and Techniques for Tax Technicians* (Cat. No. IRM 4 [12] 20), $1.50.

For professional persons, the publication entitled *Audit Technique Handbook for Internal Revenue Agents* is probably better. It contains fairly detailed discussions of ways to investigate persons in certain professions, such as medicine and law. Its catalog number is IRM 4231 and it costs $2.25.

Both publications are available from the Freedom of Information Reading Room, Room 1565, Internal Revenue Service, 1111 Constitution Avenue N.W., Washington, D.C. 20224.

If you're interested in the workings of the IRS, you will get a broader picture by spending $7.50 for a year's subscription to *People & Taxes*. The monthly newspaper on taxes is published by Public Citizen, P.O. Box 14198, Washington, D.C. 20004.

What You Should Know about Discount Stockbrokers

The small investor's enthusiasm for the stock market is, at best, inconstant. From time to time a wave of speculative fever washes over people who would in cooler moments keep their money in savings and other stable investments. The wave typically recedes when these same investors, having bought during a period of rising stock prices, discover that prices fall as well as rise.

Since 1970, the tide's been going out. The New York Stock Exchange reports that from 1970 to 1975 the number of individual stockholders declined by 5.6 million to 25.3 million, a drop of 18 percent. The largest decline was among young shareholders between the ages of twenty-one and forty-four.

Undoubtedly, the relentless erosion of stock prices during the long market decline of the early 1970s was the major reason that people sought more secure investments, such as savings accounts or time deposits. But another factor was the high commission cost of buying and selling stock—a sometimes overlooked cost that can turn a small paper profit into a dollars-and-cents loss.

Until recently, investors had little reason to shop for low commission rates. All major brokers charged about the same fees. Brokerage rates for trades on the New York Stock Exchange (where most trades take place) were figured according to a rigid minimum-rate schedule set by the stock exchange. But in May 1975, the Securities and Exchange Commission (SEC) abolished the minimum-rate schedule and decreed that rates would henceforth be subject to negotiation between brokers and investors. The idea was to establish a competitive rate structure.

Competition has worked out just fine for institutional investors, such as banks, insurance companies, and pension funds, which have been able to negotiate sizable discounts from the old fixed-rate schedule. But it hasn't worked out nearly so well for small investors—those who trade in blocks of two hundred shares or less.

An SEC study shows that brokerage rates for these investors, who place most of the individual orders, actually increased by 2 percent from April 1975 to March 1976, while commission rates for institutions doing comparable business decreased by 23 percent. Large institutions have been able to negotiate discounts of as much as 85 percent. The typical small investor pays a commission of about fifty-one cents per share while large institutions have been able to haggle their commission rates down to ten or twelve cents per share.

The difference is large enough so that, as small investors regain an interest in a recovering stock market, they might also want to consider making their transactions through discount commission brokers—bare-bones operations that dispense with fancy offices, research analysts, and sales personnel and simply execute the orders of their customers.

To see what the saving might be on a typical transaction, we queried some large brokerage houses and some discount brokers about the costs of buying one round lot (100 shares) of a $30 stock. (We chose a $30 stock because that was about the average price of a share traded on the New York Stock Exchange in spring 1976.) The commissions for buying 100 shares of that stock ranged from a high of about $59 at Merrill Lynch, Pierce, Fenner & Smith, Bache Halsey Stuart, and Dean Witter & Co., three of the largest brokerage houses, to a low of $23 at Burke, Christensen & Lewis Securities, Inc., a Chicago discounter. (For more information on brokers' commissions, see the table below.)

What It Costs to Trade Stocks

The table below gives the ranges of commission rates charged for four typical stocks by three of the country's largest brokerage houses and by eight discount brokers. New York State transfer tax and SEC fees are not included. Commission prices, rounded to the nearest dollar, are as of mid-August 1976.

	$30 Stock		$50 Stock	
	Commission on 50 shares	Commission on 100 shares	Commission on 50 shares	Commission on 100 shares
Large Brokerage Houses	$26-$40	$47-$59	$42-$54	$68-$82
Discounters	$23-$30	$23-$43	$23-$40	$23-$60

It should be noted that not all brokerage houses go out of their way to make their charges clear. When CU tried to learn about commission rates, we found Merrill Lynch, Bache Halsey, and Dean Witter more than cooperative. (We called their headquarters for commission rates on specific transactions, and then called brokers in a few branch offices at random, to check the information we received.)

But we had some difficulty when we contacted E. F. Hutton & Co., whose commercials proclaim, "when E. F. Hutton talks, people listen." The problem, we found, is getting the firm to talk. The company's spokesperson declined to tell us what rates the firm charged on a variety of transactions. A broker at one of its branch offices refused to give a CU staffer any information on rates unless he could be assured an order would result. Brokers in two other E. F. Hutton offices did quote rates—but different rates for the same trades.

We found discount brokers more than willing to explain how they figure their rates and to quote the cost of a given transaction. But some discount brokers don't want to be bothered with stock-market neophytes. "If you just inherited $7,000 worth of stock from your aunt and simply want to sell it, you should go to a place like Merrill Lynch," says Jeffrey W. Casdin, president of Source Securities of New York, one of the largest discounters. "Our typical customer has at least $10,000 of risk money and likes to work his account month in and month out." Other firms have different philosophies. Lawrence H. Weiss, president of Odd Lots Securities Ltd., another New York discounter, says his firm's typical customer "invests $1,000 or so, four times a year."

The discounters have one thing in common, though. They cater to people who can make up their own minds about what stocks to buy and sell and when to buy and sell them. None of the discounters give investment advice; they are neither equipped for nor interested in assisting the person who relies on the advice of a stockbroker for investment decisions.

To do business with a discount broker, you phone your order into a trading desk, which buys or sells the stocks you want and later confirms the trade by mail. Most brokers have toll-free 800 numbers or accept collect calls. By "settlement day" (five business days after the transaction), you must either send the firm a check for the securities you bought or deliver the stock certificates of the securities you sold.

It's not unusual for a discounter to ask a new customer to put down all or some of the cash required for the first buy order, or to furnish the stock certificates before the first sell order. Some firms, interested in serving only active customers who trade frequently, require new customers to pay a certain amount of commissions in advance. Source Securities, for instance, requires an advance of $250, which is then credited against commissions subsequently generated by the customer. Kingsley Boye & Southwood, a broker that has just entered the discount business, charges a $150 annual service fee *in addition to commissions*.

Most discounters (like some large brokerage firms) have a minimum fee per transaction, which tends to discourage orders under $1,000 or so. The minimums range from $15 to $30, with most between $20 and $25.

Discounters have two basic methods of figuring commission rates. Most discount from the old New York Stock Exchange schedule. The smaller the transaction, the smaller the discount. Discounts often begin at 10 or 20 percent off and rise to a maximum of 50 percent off (sometimes very large orders can command discounts of as much as 75 percent or so). Others charge a flat fee per share plus a minimum fee per trade, usually 8½ cents per share plus $25. Some firms charge extra for delivering stock certificates to their customers, and others charge a higher commission for "limit" orders (orders to buy or sell a stock at a specific price, rather than at the prevailing market price).

Many discounters have a two-tier pricing system: a

higher commission rate for trades executed on the major stock exchanges and a lower rate for trades in the so-called third market. The third market isn't really a physical marketplace at all, but a network of traders who bypass the major stock exchanges and buy and sell stocks listed on the exchanges among themselves. Some brokers claim there's a "hidden charge" in the third market because prices obtained for securities there aren't always as good as prices obtained on the floor of the New York Stock Exchange. That's a difficult charge to prove, however, and minute price differences really don't amount to much for small investors, who may deal in no more than 50 or 100 shares.

Actually, it's more likely that some consumers pay a "hidden charge" simply because they are small investors. Amivest Corp., a Wall Street research firm, has studied the way various brokerage houses execute trades for large institutions. It found that although the prestige and size of a brokerage house does not necessarily equate with the firm's quality of execution, there is one common denominator: Small orders (those between 100 and 500 shares) consistently receive "poor treatment," regardless of the type or size of brokerage firm handling the trade. Michael D. Hirsch, a vice president of Amivest, said it's likely that individuals placing small orders receive "equally poor treatment." If you can't be assured of top-quality execution at a big-name firm or a little-known one, then it would seem logical to place your order at the firm where the costs are lowest.

Aside from reduced commission rates, a few discounters reward investors who leave funds on deposit with the brokers by paying interest on these funds, called *free credit balances*. Brown & Co. of Boston pays 5 percent on balances above $2,000, while Charles Schwab & Co., San Francisco, places the funds in a savings and loan association that pays

5¼ percent on all balances higher than $100.

Discount brokers don't offer the only opportunity for small investors to cut commission costs, however. Consumers who live in large cities may be able to save by placing their orders through the banks where they maintain checking or savings accounts. Large banks usually maintain stock-trading desks for their own purposes. Often, they'll act as agents for their regular customers who want to buy or sell securities. The banks use their institutional muscle to negotiate low commission rates for themselves and pass on these low rates to their customers. Even though the banks sometimes tack on a service fee of $20 or $25 to cover their own costs, consumers are generally better off than they would be if they went to a large brokerage house.

Chemical Bank in New York, for instance, charges $25 in addition to a commission rate of ten cents per share. So a 100-share order of that hypothetical $30 stock mentioned earlier would cost $35, compared with $59 at Merrill Lynch. (Chemical is also promoting a similar arrangement in a test program but charging customers an additional $30 annual "membership" fee to cover promotional and administrative expenses.) Our research indicates that other banks in New York, Philadelphia, Chicago, and California also buy and sell stocks for customers, though costs vary.

The trick is to find out whether your bank offers such a service. Many of the bank officials we spoke with were unaware that such arrangements existed at their institutions. That's probably because the service isn't promoted, since banks regard it only as an accommodation for their regular customers. If the manager of your local branch doesn't know whether your bank offers such a service, find out if the bank has a trader and direct your inquiries to that person.

Discount brokers are particularly attractive to traders—

people who buy and sell fairly frequently in the hope of realizing more dramatic gains than they would expect by holding stock for long periods. Consumers who don't have the interest or money needed to "play the market" but who nevertheless want to accumulate stock slowly might consider one of the special investment programs offered by some of the large brokerage houses. Merrill Lynch's Sharebuilder plan, which offers discounts of 15 to 40 percent on trades below $5,000 is favored by the National Association of Investment Clubs. Under the plan, consumers must first send in their money or stock certificates. Their trades are not executed until the market opens on the morning following arrival of the cash or securities, and limit orders are not accepted. Bache Halsey has a somewhat similar program called Stockinvest (it covers only fifty stocks and trades are executed only twice a month) and Paine, Webber, Jackson & Curtis has one called Econo-Trade. Some commercial banks offer similar arrangements, known as automatic stock investment plans or dividend reinvestment programs.

Sometimes consumers who are trying to sell a few shares of a high-priced stock run into problems because brokers are reluctant to handle a small one-time transaction at any price. This is particularly troublesome for people who have acquired fairly expensive securities under stock-purchase plans sponsored by corporate employers. An IBM credit union in Westchester County, N.Y., has solved the problem by acting as an agent for its members, pooling their sales orders and placing the trade with a third-market firm. The cost is far less than with a large broker. While the idea is apparently still unique, we think it's one that other large credit unions could well copy.

Buying a House? How to Deal with Closing Costs

Few American families can afford to buy their dream house these days. In fact, a 1975 report by the Congressional Joint Economic Committee found that it takes an annual income of about $23,000 to afford an average new house—and only one family in six earns that much. Whether you scrape together enough for a new house, settle for an older one, or sell the house you already own to buy another, there's still one more financial hurdle to jump: closing costs.

In most parts of the country, these one-time costs come due at the time of the house closing—the meeting at which the buyer signs the mortgage papers, turns over the proceeds to the seller, and obtains the title to the property. (In most Western states, the parties deposit signed papers and any money due with an escrow agent, and no formal meeting is held.) The charges for the numerous closing services may be small individually, but they can add up to a large bill —and a big shock—to the unprepared homebuyer. Closing, or settlement, costs include attorneys' fees and charges for items such as title search, title insurance, loan processing, credit reports, and surveys. At the closing, the buyer must also pay an adjustment for real estate taxes, plus certain other government fees.

Depending on where you live, where you get your mortgage loan, and how you handle the closing, total costs on closing day can range from just under 1 percent of a house's sales price to nearly 7 percent—or anywhere from about \$350 to about \$2,450 on a \$35,000 house.

In the past, the shock usually didn't come until the actual closing day, when the buyer, on cue from an attorney, wrote check after check. In June 1975, the Real Estate Settlement Procedures Act (RESPA) went into effect. It required the mortgage-lender in most cases to itemize and disclose the estimated settlement costs at least twelve days before closing. It also required lenders to give consumers at the time they apply for a loan a copy of *Settlement Costs*, a useful information booklet on closing costs, and to provide buyers with a uniform settlement statement that lists buyer and seller expenses side by side.

As a result of lobbying on the part of real estate interests and the financial community connected with real estate, Congress took another look at RESPA and modified the law. As of June 30, 1976, when a buyer applies for a loan the lender must give the buyer, along with the copy of *Settlement Costs*, a nonbinding, "good faith" estimate of most of the closing charges, either in terms of a specific dollar amount or as a price range. Then, with a few exceptions, upon the request of the buyer the lender is obliged, one business day before the settlement, to show the buyer all of the relevant information available. Under the original version of RESPA the buyer had a little more advance notice of the amount needed for closing costs—and more time to collect the money—as well as an outside chance to get a better deal through comparison shopping and negotiation. But even with the watered-down version of the law, the shock of closing costs might be lessened somewhat.

The Department of Housing and Urban Development (HUD) studied some fifty thousand closing transactions across the country and analyzed closing practices in thirteen metropolitan areas in 1971. The study found striking differences from one place to the next in the kind of closing fees that were charged, who paid for them, and how much they amounted to. The costs varied within geographic areas as well as among regions of the country. They were highest in metropolitan areas of the Middle Atlantic states, where both title insurance and attorneys are involved in most transactions. Closing costs were far lower in the New England states and the northern Plains states, where independent abstractors or attorneys conduct the title search, and where title insurance and surveys are little used.

In 1974, Senator William Proxmire updated the 1971 HUD figures and found that the national average for closing costs was $860, even without adjustments for real estate taxes and special assessments. The average varied from state to state, ranging from a low of $476 in South Dakota to a high of $1,278 in New York.

The HUD study also found wide variations in the manner of closing and who footed the bill for it. In Newark, N.J., where the buyer pays for title insurance, the title documents are frequently reviewed by attorneys for the buyer and the lender—and the buyer pays for both lawyers. In Washington, D.C., where title companies do most of the work, attorneys are rarely retained by the buyer or seller. In Chicago, the seller, not the buyer, customarily pays for the title insurance report, preparation of the deed, and the state transfer tax. In Los Angeles, where the closing on a house is taken care of by neutral escrow companies, the buyer and the seller split the escrow fee.

Practices vary so widely that it's hard to generalize about what specific charges homebuyers will encounter. The best way to keep settlement costs to a minimum is to become familiar with the types of fees likely to be charged, even though some may not be charged in your community or by your lender.

There are four basic categories of costs that homebuyers must pay at the closing:

1. **Attorneys' fees.** In many parts of the country, it's customary for a homebuyer to retain a lawyer to review the contract of sale and the loan and real estate documents and to handle the closing. Sometimes one attorney represents seller, buyer, and lender (although there are serious questions about the ethics of such an arrangement). Sometimes the buyer must pay for lawyers representing various parties to the transaction. In Western states, title and escrow companies often do this work.

2. **Loan charges.** In addition to interest, this category includes fees charged by lenders for putting the mortgage loan on the books and for such miscellaneous items as credit reports and preparing documents.

3. **Title examination and title insurance.** A title examination is a search of records of previous ownership to establish that the seller actually owns the property and that it is free from legal claims that could cloud the buyer's title. The search is conducted by a lawyer, a professional investigator known as an abstractor, or a title company, depending on local practice. Title insurance insures lenders (and buyers if they pay an extra fee) against any loss from errors in the title search and from certain problems that can't be discovered by a search. Lenders usually require title insurance before they will extend a mortgage loan.

4. **Taxes and government fees.** These include the buyer's

share of the property taxes and special assessments already paid for the entire year by the seller, as well as any state or local taxes imposed when property changes hands or when a mortgage is given.

Attorneys' Fees

If the only attorney involved in the closing represents the lender, bear in mind that the attorney places the lender's interest first—even though you may pay the bill. Although legal fees are kept to a minimum when a single attorney handles the paperwork for both buyer and lender, it may be difficult to find an attorney to adequately represent your personal interest in such a situation. If local custom is for one attorney to represent both the buyer and the lender at the closing, ask the lender if *you* can designate the attorney. That may improve the objectivity of the legal counsel you receive.

If the lender refuses, you may wish to retain an attorney just to review the sales contract, which sets forth the terms of the house purchase. Retain your attorney early on—after you find the house but before you sign anything—whether it's a personal check or a receipt torn from a real estate broker's pad. Don't wait until the closing, because by that time you will have committed yourself to a deal the attorney can only rubber-stamp. You'll get the greatest value for your legal dollars by having your attorney at your side during the crucial negotiations over the language of the sales contract. (See page 105 for a discussion of some of the provisions the ideal sales contract should contain.) You might also want your own attorney to review the proposed loan papers before you commit yourself to a particular mortgage loan.

If this is your first house, or if you don't feel comfortable without professional legal advice, you may wish to retain your own lawyer for the entire transaction. The attorney would then negotiate the sales contract, review the title report, and represent you at the closing. This may mean you will pay two sizable legal fees : one to your lawyer and another to the lender's lawyer. And in some areas it may be difficult for you to find a lawyer competent in real estate matters who does not also represent the lender or the title company in your transaction.

Traditionally, attorneys have charged homebuyers according to "minimum fee schedules" drawn up by state or local bar associations. The charges under these schedules were based largely on the sales price of the house rather than on the work actually performed. In June 1975, the United States Supreme Court ruled that uniform fee schedules for title examinations constitute a form of illegal price-fixing in violation of antitrust laws. The high court's decision has opened the door for competitive pricing by lawyers, and it's likely that fees for this type of work will be reduced. (In Fairfax County, Va., where the suit was brought, many lawyers have already cut their title-examination fees by as much as 50 percent.)

In the new environment created by the Supreme Court ruling, CU believes the best way to keep legal costs down is to ask the lawyer to bill you at an hourly rate for work actually performed. Ask for an estimate of the time involved and the total bill before you go ahead. You may wish to question a few attorneys about their rates before you finally select one. Don't be shy about suggesting a lower fee ; young attorneys just starting practice or established ones who want your other legal business may be quite willing to adjust their fees downward.

A helpful booklet called the *Homebuyer's Checklist* outlines some of the legal pitfalls that confront prospective buyers. It's available for $1 from the National Homebuyers and Homeowners Association, 1225 19th Street, N.W., Washington, D.C. 20036.

Loan Charges

Contact lenders well before you've found your house—even before you've started to look. If you plan on buying a house within the next six months or so, visit a savings bank or savings and loan association (S&L) and tell the mortgage officer you'll deposit your savings at the bank in return for an indication that your future mortgage needs will get special consideration. (Since interest rates can fluctuate sharply, it's unlikely you'll be guaranteed a specific interest rate; but such a commitment will at least improve your access to mortgage money if funds get tight, assuming there's no difficulty with your credit standing or with the property involved.) If the officer hems and haws, take your business elsewhere.

When you've finally found a house, compare the rates and charges at your own bank or S&L (at that point, the loan officer should be willing to quote you a specific interest rate) with those of competing institutions. First, ask about the total terms of financing—the amount of the down payment required and the annual percentage rate of interest (see page 10). Sometimes, the larger the down payment, the lower the annual percentage rate.

But there are some other potential costs you should consider before choosing a lender. Chief among them is an *origination fee* charged by some institutions. This fee, normally 1 percent or more of the face amount of the mortgage (it would equal $350 on a $35,000 mortgage), supposedly compensates lenders for the cost of processing the loan and helps maintain their profit should you pay off the loan early.

If you are charged an origination fee, you should not also be subject to a *prepayment penalty*, which allows the lender to collect an extra charge if you repay the loan ahead of time, as you may well wish to do if you later sell the house. Try to avoid either charge; strenuously resist allowing both to be written into the final mortgage contract.

Lenders frequently charge *miscellaneous fees* for such items as loan applications, credit reports, notary service, preparing papers, reviewing papers prepared by others, and the actual settlement meeting. CU believes you should not be charged such fees in addition to a loan origination fee, which should more than cover those items. If no origination fee is assessed, pay close attention to these extra charges and tally up the total for comparison with other banks' fees.

Lenders often require an *appraisal* of the house and a *survey* of the property before they grant the loan, and they charge for them. An appraisal is something a buyer may want in any case, to help negotiate a fair price with the seller. But sometimes the lender will refuse to give the buyer a copy of the appraisal report. We believe that if you won't receive a copy of the appraisal report, it's unreasonable for the lender to charge you for it.

A survey may also be a superfluous expense. If the seller has a survey no more than five years old and has made no major changes to the property, ask the lender to accept it rather than put you to the expense of a new one. That could save you from $75 to $250. If the survey is older, ask if the seller will sign an affidavit of "no change," swearing there have been no major changes made since the survey was conducted. If the lender insists on an updated survey, ask if a "visual inspection" will do; that's much less expensive than a full-scale survey with stakes and markers. (You can try to rate-shop among surveyors, but we're not too hopeful that it will get you anywhere. A pamphlet distributed by a surveyors' trade association says bidding for work on the basis of fees "should be discouraged.")

Title Examination and Title Insurance

Before lenders will extend a loan on a house, they want assurances that the seller has the legal right to transfer the property and that there are no hidden claims or liens filed against it. This entails a meticulous search through various documents in the public records.

The searcher combs the records of previous ownership to be sure the owners paid off their mortgages and any other claims against the property, such as income or inheritance taxes. The HUD report noted that searchers had to check sixteen different government offices and about eighty different types of records before they could certify a clear title. (In some states, even dog-tax records must be checked.)

The title search can be time-consuming, since all the relevant records are rarely located in the same place. Because of the decentralized (and often disorganized) way land records are kept, a title search is a cumbersome and costly step in the transfer of property, and a step that must be repeated each time the property is sold. (Simpler and cheaper alternatives are possible; see page 97 for a discussion of some of them.)

There's always the chance that even the most thorough title search will fail to uncover a claim and that the claimant could file an expensive lawsuit against the new owners and eventually even wrest the property from them. For example, a past deed might have been forged or signed by a minor and therefore may not have legally conveyed the title. Or the spouse or heirs of a former owner might not have given up their interest in the real estate when that owner sold it. Or the records themselves might be improperly filed or they might be indexed incorrectly.

Title insurance was developed to protect lenders against

losses from such situations. But such losses are rare. A study by the American Land Title Association, the industry trade group, found that losses and loss adjustment expense in 1973—although the highest since the group began collecting the data—came to only 5.3 percent of the title companies' operating income. A 1971 study by Senator Proxmire found the risk absorbed by these companies was "almost nonexistent." That's not surprising, since title companies are in the business of avoiding risk by meticulous searches rather than assuming it. In fact, the premium for title insurance is based only partially on risk; it's calculated on the sales price of the house and the amount of the mortgage. Unlike premiums for other insurance, the premium for title insurance is paid only once, rather than at regular intervals over a period of time.

The *national rate* for title insurance to protect the lender (the rate for the insurance alone, without a title search) is $2.50 per thousand dollars of mortgage. In 1975, for a house with a $35,000 mortgage, that amounted to $87.50— not terribly expensive. The problem is that many con sumers can't buy title insurance at the national rate. Instead they must either pay a lawyer to search the title or pay the *company examination rate* (the rate for a title search *and* title insurance). The combined rate is double or even triple the charge for insurance alone. In the Westchester County suburbs of New York City, the company examination rate for a house with a $35,000 mortgage would be $205; in Jacksonville, Fla., the cost would be $287.50.

It's hard to believe that the title company's own cost of searching a title is as high as the charge for the company examination rate would indicate. One New York title company told CU that it farms out its searches to low-paid freelancers, and the cost runs anywhere from $30 to $55. A summary of the search, called an abstract, is turned over to the company, where it is normally reviewed in forty-five minutes or so. The company's internal cost for such a search under this procedure seems much lower than $117.50, which is the difference between the company examination rate ($205) and the national rate ($87.50).

One contributor to the high combined cost of title protection has been the commissions that title companies have paid to lawyers and real estate brokers who steered homebuyers to them. The commissions—kickbacks, actually—ranged from 15 to 25 percent of the premium, depending on the company and the state. Under RESPA, such payments are no longer legal unless some service is performed for the commission. It remains to be seen, however, if title costs will come down, since the law doesn't require the title companies to reduce their premiums by the amount of the commissions they are no longer permitted to pay. (New York State has passed such a law. In response, title companies asked the New York State Insurance Department for a rate increase of over 40 percent. All but one company received a 16 percent rate increase; that one received less because its rates were already higher than the others.)

Land Transfers and Title Insurance

When it comes to real estate sales, the United States is "unique in its backwardness and is just plain underdeveloped," says Barlow Burke, Jr., a professor at American University Law School and one of the authors of an analysis of closing costs done by HUD.

The current system of storing land records descends directly from Colonial times, when land changed hands infrequently and most property was in the hands of the original owners or their recent heirs. As the turnover rate increased, so did the potential for record-keeping errors. Title searchers today must check in one place through volumes of past property owners; thumb through files of mort-gage-lenders in another place; inspect inheritance-tax records somewhere else; and on and on. The growing number of these records has far outstripped the ability of local governments to deal with them. In many areas public records are kept so poorly that title companies maintain their own versions of these documents.

Such an unwieldy, disorganized system of land records makes title insurance a virtual necessity in many areas of the country. But the system can be simplified and the costs reduced, as demonstrated by the experience in other countries and in some parts of the United States. For years, concerned lawyers have urged that we replace our agrarian system of dealing with land records with a modernized one more suited to the needs of a mobile urban society. The basic system of real estate titles and transfers "cries out for reexamination and simplification," says Chief Justice Warren E. Burger. Here are some of the most frequently discussed recommendations for reform.

1. Adopt a Torrens-like system. Named for an Australian public official who applied a method of registering ships to registering real property, this system simplifies the process of establishing a clear title. Under a Torrens system, the title to real property is registered once and remains permanently on file for inspection, in much the same way as the title to your car does. By contrast, under the United States system, only the individual documents (deeds, mortgages, etc.) relating to a title are registered.

A Torrens title shows the exact current status of the land; matters affecting it are added to the original document. If a defect in the title does not appear on the face of the certificate, then it does not legally exist so far as the buyer is concerned. The Torrens system eliminates the need for a full-blown search every time the property is sold.

A person with a claim against the title has no claim against the actual property under a Torrens system. Legitimate claims are instead satisfied by a monetary award from a public insurance fund, which is financed by imposing a special recording fee when the land is registered under the Torrens system for the first time.

Torrens-like systems are in use in England, Canada, and Israel. Limited versions of Torrens systems are also in effect in parts of the United States—notably Boston, Chicago, and Minneapolis-St. Paul. The costs of transferring property under such a system can be far less than the costs with title insurance. In Chicago, for instance, one can transfer title to a house already registered under the Torrens system, without using an attorney, for only $28. The cost to bring a new $45,000 house within the system would typically be about $118.

But less than one-third of all parcels in the Chicago area are "Torrenized." Why? The HUD study noted that one title company, Chicago Title & Trust, controls 90 percent of the business in the area (it's the only company with records from before the 1871 Chicago fire). According to the study, some developers said they'd been offered greatly reduced title rates in return for a promise not to use the Torrens system. In addition, many lenders (who frequently hold directorships on title company boards) require title insurance even on properties registered under the Torrens system. Such opposition from those who profit from expensive searches is one major reason why Torrens systems have not made more headway in the United States.

2. **Modernize land records** and keep them together so that they can be easily retrieved. Do away with alphabetical name indexes, which relate the records to the names of past and present owners, and file most documents by means of tract indexes, which relate the records to the property.

Require the use of "land parcel identifiers," which are geographically coded to reflect a property's unique position on the earth's surface. One section of RESPA authorized HUD to test methods of modernizing title records. Many experts consider this one of the most important sections of the bill. But HUD hasn't requested any funds for testing.

3. **Enact "marketable title" acts,** which allow title to property to be determined by a search of recent records, not ancient ones. HUD found that states with such legislation had "significantly lower" costs than states without.

4. **Make lenders pay for settlement services** they require, such as title search and insurance, credit reports, surveys, and appraisals. Collectively, these institutions have much more economic leverage than individual homebuyers and presumably they would be able to negotiate lower charges. Such an arrangement would also give them a greater incentive to cut costs. While this approach would probably result in a slight increase in mortgage interest rates, at least the higher cost could be amortized over the life of the entire loan, and buyers could write off some of the cost as an income-tax deduction.

How to Shop for Title Insurance

Expensive title insurance is not the only way to protect against title claims. Indeed, as we've said, in some parts of the country, buyers and lenders get along nicely without it. But until the system is reformed, most homebuyers will have no option. So here's what you should know about what you're buying—and what you're not buying:

First, as previously noted, the premium most homebuyers pay for title insurance protects the lender, not the homebuyer. If you want to cover yourself, you must specifically ask for an *owner's policy* (also known as a "fee" policy). If you buy an owner's policy, purchase it at the same time you buy the lender's policy, and ask for a *simultaneous policy*. The rate for the two policies purchased in tandem is considerably lower than the rate for the two policies if purchased separately. A simultaneous policy for a $45,000 house with a $35,000 mortgage in Jacksonville would cost about $409, while an owner's and lender's policy bought separately would cost $625.

Is title insurance for the buyer worth the money, considering the minuscule risk of claims against the house? The housing authorities interviewed by CU generally think it is, since a house is probably the most important and expensive purchase a consumer will make. "A serious title defect may occur only once in every ten thousand cases," according to Dale A. Whitman, professor of law at Brigham Young University and a consultant to HUD on closing costs, "but when it happens the effect can be devastating."

No matter what kind of title policy you decide to buy, you can try to shop for the lowest title premiums available. Sometimes a firm that is just entering an area will cut prices to attract business, and the HUD study did find striking cost variations. But in a number of states, title companies belong to "rating bureaus," which fix prices by filing uniform rates with the state insurance department. Such collusion would appear to fly in the face of U.S. antitrust laws, and, in fact, the Federal Trade Commission is investigating the title-insurance industry for this very reason.

In 1975, CU shoppers did some checking in Florida, New York, and Pennsylvania. They called ten different title companies in these states and asked for "simultaneous rates" on a hypothetical $45,000 house. Here were the results: the three companies in Westchester County, N.Y., all charged $336; the three companies in Philadelphia County, Pa., all charged $378; and the four companies in

Duval County, Fla., all charged $409.

The New York State Department of Insurance wasn't much help. When a CU shopper called to ask for aid in finding the least expensive title company, a clerk stated that the department would "certainly not help consumers comparison shop . . . but a mutual company usually has the lowest rates." (There is only one mutual title-insurance company that we know of.) The clerk hung up when the shopper attempted to question him further. A higher-level official later apologized for the misinformation and the brush-off but added he would refer consumers seeking price information to the local rating bureau—which, of course, files uniform rates with the state insurance department.

If the house you are buying has been insured by a title company recently (within the past two to ten years), you may be eligible for a reduced rate, called a *reissue rate*. The discount can range from 5 to 40 percent, depending on the company and how long ago it first insured the property.

Reissue rates are not usually publicized. Ask about them; this is an area where asking questions can save a substantial amount of money. Of the four companies we called in the Jacksonville area, one offered a reissue discount of $135; a second, a discount of $84; a third, a discount of $74; and a fourth, no discount at all. Don't expect the companies to volunteer discount information routinely, though; two of the Florida companies told CU that reissue rates were "something we seldom get asked about," and it took them a while to figure out what their reissue rates were.

Sometimes there are differences among company policies, even though companies may charge the same rates. If you buy an owner's policy, ask for the latest policy distributed by the American Land Title Association, called ALTA form B-1970. That form is more favorable to consumers than earlier ALTA forms or the forms of any of the various state title-company associations.

You or your attorney should insist that the seller remove some of the *exceptions* to insurance coverage that appear on Schedule B of the title-insurance form. Sometimes called the objection page, this is the most important part of the entire policy; it lists items the insurance will not cover. You can ask for a copy a week or two before closing and review it as part of a "preliminary title report." Most of the exceptions on Schedule B are negotiable.

First, look at any exceptions that have been typed in. These may include the first mortgage still owed by the seller. It should be paid off—and stricken as an exception—at the time of closing.

Other exceptions may be in the form of restrictive covenants, which limit what you can do with and on the property. Such covenants may prohibit raising farm animals on the land or selling alcoholic beverages—things you normally would not want to do anyway in a residential neighborhood. But such covenants could also restrict the type of architecture permitted for new dwellings.

Finally, the typed-in exceptions may include easements that allow a town or a utility company to come onto your land to maintain such things as drainage ditches or telephone lines. Be sure you understand what these easements mean and how they may affect your future plans for the land. (You may, for instance, intend to install a swimming pool where a town drainage ditch now exists.)

You should also try to get some standard printed exceptions removed. One exception won't cover "the rights of parties in possession of the property but not shown on the public records." Yet this type of claim is precisely what title insurance is supposed to insure against. Many title companies will remove this exception at the closing, if asked. Matters "which would be disclosed by an accurate survey" are sometimes listed as another standard exception. This is a reasonable procedure if you haven't obtained a survey; but if you have, insist on having this exception removed.

Another standard exception won't cover mechanics' liens, that is, claims against real estate filed by persons who previously did work on a house but weren't paid for it; such liens could eventually result in foreclosure of the property to settle the debt. Mechanics' liens are particularly troublesome because they can be filed a number of months after the work was completed and thus may not show up on a title search. The amount can be substantial if, for example, the seller did extensive remodeling to put the house in shape for sale, or if it's a new house with subcontractors' bills still outstanding. Then the stakes are high enough to warrant trying to get that exception removed.

In many states, the method of removing a mechanics' lien exception is to purchase an "endorsement." In Philadelphia in 1975, for example, the cost of this endorsement varied and could range up to a maximum of $5 per thousand dollars of the house's selling price—or $225 more for a $45,000 house. One title company representative told CU that this is one area where comparison shopping can uncover some significant price differences.

Taxes and Government Fees

Adjustments of certain costs, such as real estate taxes and special assessments for such municipal improvements as sewers, are prorated so that the sellers are charged for the period they owned the property and the buyers for the period after settlement.

Transfer taxes are assessed when property changes hands or when a mortgage loan is granted. There's not much room for negotiation here, since these charges are imposed by state law (although you can try to get the seller to split the costs with you). In addition, fees are generally charged for recording documents with government offices. There's a wide variation from one state to another in the size of these charges. The HUD study found they ranged from a low of .05 percent of a house's selling price in Wyoming to a high of more than 2 percent in Maryland.

Sometimes lenders require you to place money in an "escrow" or "impound" account in order to accumulate funds for future payment of taxes and fire-insurance premiums. RESPA puts a limit on the amount a lender can demand per month and on the amount that has to be put into the account at closing, but it does not require lenders to pay interest to consumers on the money. Some Eastern states, such as New York and Connecticut, do require lenders to pay interest on escrow accounts—but the minimum interest rate is usually well below the typical savings passbook rate. If a lender refuses to pay the passbook rate of interest, try to get the escrow requirement waived so you can pay your own taxes and insurance. Or give the lender the right to dip into your savings account (if you save at the bank or S&L that holds your mortgage), should you fail to make your tax and insurance payments on time.

The Sales Contract

The cardinal rule in buying a house is: Don't hurry. This is probably the most expensive and important purchase of your life, and you may regret rushing into it without careful consideration. It's worth repeating that if you plan to retain an attorney, the time to do so is after you've found the house you want but before you've put your signature to a personal check, a receipt for the real estate broker, or any piece of paper.

Normally, the first step is to make what is called an

"earnest-money" or "binder" deposit. The amount of this deposit is determined by custom, not law, and can range from $50 or $100 to as much as 10 percent of the sales price. The amount is negotiable; try to put down as little as possible. Regardless of the amount, don't turn over any money unless you've decided to buy the house. An earnest-money deposit is an offer to buy the property at a specific price, and if the offer is accepted it may be impossible for you to back out of the deal without suffering financially.

Ask for a receipt that states the price you are willing to pay for the house and gives a termination date for the offer. (Normally, the seller is allowed five to seven days to decide whether or not to accept an offer.) In some parts of the country, the earnest-money transaction is separate from the actual sales contract, which is drawn up only after the offer is accepted. In other areas of the country, the earnest-money receipt contains the complete contract of sale, and no further contract will be signed. Either way, you will be signing something that could be binding, so it's essential that your lawyer review the language of any document before you turn over the earnest money.

Any earnest-money receipt should state that the deposit money is totally refundable if the offer is refused. To protect you in the event the offer is accepted but you decide to back out, the receipt should also state that the sellers can retain only that portion of the deposit that compensates them for any losses they may incur, and that any excess must be returned to you.

The sales contract sets forth the terms of the property purchase. A contract that provides the buyer with maximum protection should include the following provisions, even if they're not standard.

1. Contract contingent on buyer obtaining acceptable financing. The contract should spell out the type of mortgage

loan (conventional or government-insured), the minimum amount of the loan, the maximum annual percentage rate of interest, and the minimum term.

2. Contract contingent on buyer approval of the title report. Obtain a copy of the title report from the title company or abstractor and read it carefully, with special attention to the exceptions listed on Schedule B of the policy form (see page 101). If there are any exceptions to insurance coverage you do not understand or agree with, ask for an explanation or try to get the exceptions removed.

3. "Time is of the essence" clause. Normally, the law says the exact date for closing in a contract is not binding, but this clause ensures a firm closing date. If you think you might have trouble arranging financing by the closing date or need to sell your present house first, add an extension clause giving you the option to postpone the closing for a stated period. With a new house, it's especially important to have a firm completion date, as well as a penalty clause that states that in the event completion is delayed, the builder will pay you a certain amount per diem for motel accommodations until the house is ready. The builder will probably resist, but it's a point that is still worth bargaining for.

4. Seller pays for title examination and title insurance. Even if this is not local practice, try anyway; there's no law against it. If the seller won't pay the entire amount, perhaps you can split the cost. Try the same approach for the payment of transfer taxes.

5. Risk of loss. To protect yourself in case of serious damage, the contract should say that if there is any damage to the property beyond normal wear and tear between the signing of the contract and the closing, the price of the property will be reduced by the amount necessary to repair the damage. If the damage exceeds 5 percent of the pur-

chase price, a buyer should be able to cancel the contract.
6. Personal property and fixtures. The contract should
itemize everything included in the sales price—light fixtures, appliances, carpeting, draperies, and so on. Otherwise, you may be unpleasantly surprised when you move
into a stripped house.

7. Warranties. Have the seller warrant that the house is
in compliance with applicable building and zoning codes
and all other laws and ordinances, and have these warranties survive the settlement. (This makes the seller liable for
any problems that are not discovered until after the closing.) The seller also should warrant that the appliances and
the electrical, plumbing, heating, and air-conditioning systems are in good working order at the time of contract and
will be at the time of closing. With a new house, these "habitability" warranties should last for a certain length of
time (ideally two years, as is the case in England) and
should be transferable (should you decide to sell before that
time is up).

8. Inspections. In areas where termites are common, it is
customary for the sale to be contingent on an inspection of
the property for termites, paid for by the seller. If any ter-
mite damage is found, the seller should also bear the cost of
repair. If you are concerned about the condition of the
house's electrical and/or plumbing system, you should consider having a professional inspection of those particular
systems before signing the contract.

9. Repairs or modifications. In your negotiations, you may
wish to make the sale contingent on the completion of certain items, such as new plumbing or roofing. It may be wise
to have the escrow agent or the lender hold back a certain
portion of the purchase payment from the seller until the
repairs are completed. This is especially important with a
new house if landscaping has not yet been finished.

There are two additional areas to explore before you sign a sales contract. One concerns pending changes that could affect the neighborhood into which you are buying. Ask the local planning department if any roads, zoning changes, or nearby commercial developments are on the way.

You also need to do some investigating if the occupants of the house are not the owners. They may be tenants with a lease you will not be able to break. Again, don't depend on the word of the broker; ask the people living in the house if they have a lease, and if they do, make the sale contingent on evidence, signed by the occupants, that their lease is being terminated at the time of closing. And have the seller sign a statement that there are no outstanding leases and that the premises will be vacant at the time of the closing.

How to Reduce an Unfair Tax Assessment

For several years William Adler, a business management consultant who lives in Chicago, had been paying $2,000 a year in property taxes for his house on the city's southwest side. When he learned from a local citizen-action group that tax assessments are not always accurate or fair, he looked into his own assessment and decided to appeal it. In due course, he went before the Cook County Board of Appeals.

"They tried to bluff me out of it," Adler recalls. "They said, 'You know we can't reduce your taxes. You want services like police and fire, don't you?' " But Adler persisted; he had documented his case well and wanted to present it. Result: His assessment was reduced so much that his property taxes dropped from $2,000 to $1,200.

There are thousands of homeowners across the country who, like Adler, have learned that taxes, though inevitable, are not inevitably equitable. In July 1976, Consumers Union reported on the property-tax system and discussed the inequities that exist between the ways business property and residential property are assessed, between assessments on similar houses in neighboring communities, and between assessments on houses in the same community and even on the same street. As we've noted, the fairness of a particular assessment on a house or land is difficult for a homeowner to judge. More often than not, houses are assessed at an arbitrary fraction of market value rather than at full value. Fractional valuation can lead homeowners to believe they're underassessed, even though other assessments in town may have been set at a still lower fraction of market value.

How do such inequities come about? The fragmentation of the assessing process provides some of the answer. Only a few states, led by California, impose on their local assessment districts the strict requirements and supervision that produce a modern and reasonably equitable operation.

More typical is the situation in New York State, which assigns all authority over assessments to its localities. Some cities use computers to keep assessments up to date, aiming at 100 percent market value. Other cities stick to horse-and-buggy assessment methods that penalize some homeowners and give others big tax breaks. Qualifications for the job of assessor are not demanding. Robert Kilmer, head of New York State's Board of Equalization and Assessment, tells of a phone call he received. An assessor, elected in a rural area south of Albany, said he needed special arrangements to take the state's training course, since he was handicapped. Kilmer asked the assessor what his specific handicap was. "I can't read or write," the assessor replied.

There are three basic tax terms to understand in judging the fairness of your own taxes: appraisal, assessment, and tax rate.

An *appraisal* is a judgment of the market value of property, made either by the local assessor's office or by an appraisal firm hired by a city or town to appraise all property.

An *assessment* is the value assigned to property for tax purposes. The assessed value of the property can be the same as the appraised value, but more commonly an assessment is set at some fraction of the appraised value. When property owners appeal, it is usually on the grounds that the assessment is unfair compared with that on other similar property.

The *tax rate* is the rate applied to the assessed value in setting the property-tax figure. It's often expressed in terms of a given number of dollars per $100 or $1,000 of assessed valuation. If you are called on to pay $100 per $1,000 of assessed valuation, for example, your tax rate is 10 percent.

Few property-tax bills or assessment notices provide an understandable explanation of how to appeal, much less the data necessary to determine whether or not an assessment is fair. Yet the number of homeowners who should consider an appeal may be substantial indeed. Robert Kilmer estimates that one-third of the houses in New York State, excluding those in New York City, are assessed at more than they should be.

But the appeals process has become the preserve of professional real estate investors; relatively few homeowners bother, despite the substantial tax saving possible. A study of fifty thousand appeals in Boston over a ten-year period showed that while private homeowners owned 40 percent of the real estate, owners of apartment houses and commercial and industrial property filed 90 percent of the appeals. A study in St. Louis found that only 17 percent of appeals filed in 1974 were from private homeowners.

In this report we will describe how to find out if your

assessment is unfairly high and, if so, what you can do about it. We'll also provide some basic appeals information for each state and suggest public-interest groups that can give further help. While the procedures may sound complicated, take heart. It's quite possible to get an inequitable assessment reduced with a minimum of formality.

In Baltimore, for example, Eugene L. Jones, a real estate appraiser, decided in 1976 to appeal the assessment on his mother's house. As the first step, he asked for a copy of the assessor's worksheet, which lists the details of the house. He discovered that the worksheet incorrectly showed that the basement and attic extended beyond the actual length and width of the house. Since that and other errors overstated the size of the house by 25 percent, the assessor agreed to lower the assessment without further ado.

Across the country, in San Francisco, Dr. Richard Shadoan, a psychiatrist, appealed his assessment in 1975 partly on the grounds that houses he found comparable to his own were assessed at considerably less than his was. An appraiser sent by the assessor's office reduced the assessment by $5,000—exactly what Dr. Shadoan had asked for.

Before you can judge whether you are being fairly taxed or not, you must have a reasonably good idea of what your house is worth in today's marketplace. The easiest way to get such an estimate, of course, is to retain a professional real estate appraiser. (A professional appraiser is one who has been certified by a national organization, such as the American Institute of Real Estate Appraisers.) However, an appraisal of a house would typically cost about $100. (CU was quoted prices that ranged from $40 to $250.) A professional appraisal may be too large an investment, unless you're already sure that you can build a good case for a substantial reduction in your assessment. Some real estate agents are also certified appraisers; they might be willing to give an appraisal at a reduced fee in the hope of gaining your business should you eventually decide to sell your house. Even a real estate agent who is not a professional appraiser can make an accurate estimate of a house's market value and you might get it at no charge. But in an appeal, a professional appraisal would carry more weight.

Another way to get an estimate of market value is to find houses similar to yours that have been sold recently. Such houses are called "comparables." Try to find at least two or three houses reasonably comparable to yours—about the same size, with the same number of rooms, on a similar lot, and in the same or a similar neighborhood. Their actual selling prices would be impressive evidence of what your house is worth.

Most real estate agents receive booklets, published regularly, that list local houses for sale and record selling prices of houses that have changed hands recently. The booklets include detailed descriptions of the houses (size, number of rooms, construction, condition, lot, and so on), which make the selection of comparables possible. More than half of some twenty real estate agents CU called across the country said they would routinely make these listings available to homeowners in search of comparables.

If you can't locate a cooperative real estate agent, call a loan officer at the bank or savings and loan association that holds your mortgage. Lending institutions also receive complete records of recent sales. Some financial institutions CU called consider the records confidential; others, including two of the largest savings and loan associations in California, would permit a loan officer to aid in a search for comparables, at the loan officer's discretion.

Although it's time-consuming, you can also estimate your property's value by visiting houses advertised for sale and pricing those that are similar to yours. Since the asking price is usually higher than the price at which the transaction is made, you'll need to get some notion from the owner or agent of what an acceptable offer would be.

Once you know what your house's present market value is, you can judge whether you have grounds for appeal. Here are the appeal arguments most likely to succeed.

Your house is assessed at more than fair market value–the price you could get for the house in a normal transaction, sometimes listed as "full cash value" on property-tax bills.

Houses are usually assessed at a fraction of their market value, even in states such as New York, where the law requires assessment at full cash value. Rarely, then, is a house assessed at more than it's worth on the market. But if the assessment on your tax bill is higher than the full cash value as determined by a legitimate appraisal or by inspection of recent sales prices of comparable houses, your house has been overassessed and you should appeal.

The assessment is based on an appraisal that's too high. In taxing jurisdictions where assessments are set at some fraction of full cash value, the bill may show both the assessment and the rate of assessment. (If the bill itself does not give the rate of assessment or the assessor's judgment of full cash value, call the assessor's office and ask what the claimed rate is.) It's then a matter of simple arithmetic to arrive at the appraisal on which the assessment is based.

Thus, if your house is assessed at $20,000 and the claimed rate of assessment is 50 percent, the assessment is based on an appraisal that established full cash value at $40,000. If you can show that your house is worth only $35,000, you have grounds for an appeal–and a chance to reduce your assessment and thus your real estate taxes by 10 percent or so.

You are assessed at a greater percentage of the value of

your house than are other homeowners. Since official appraisals are sometimes deliberately low or years out of date, chances are that the appraisal on which the assessment is based is a good deal lower, not higher, than your house's cash value. That doesn't necessarily mean you're fairly assessed, however.

Suppose the houses in your community are worth an average of $50,000 and are being assessed at an average of $30,000, which would be a rate of 60 percent of full cash value. Now suppose *your* $50,000 house is assessed at $40,000, or a rate of 80 percent. Even if the assessor claims the official rate for your jurisdiction is 80, 90, or 100 percent of full cash value, the fact remains that you're assessed more strictly than average and are therefore paying more than your fair share of taxes.

But how do you find out the *rate* at which other houses are being assessed? Here you may need access to the sales prices of houses that have changed hands in recent months. If you've found a cooperative real estate agent or lending institution to help you judge comparables, you're all set. Copy down the addresses and sales prices of twenty to thirty houses that have changed hands most recently in your taxing district. (The sales prices are, of course, the best possible evidence of full cash value.) Next, visit the assessor's office and ask to inspect the assessment rolls, which list every house in the taxing district by address and give the assessment on each. (The rolls are public documents available to all citizens.) Look up the assessments for the houses on your sales list and copy down the assessments next to the selling prices.

Add up the total selling prices. Then add up the assessment figures. Divide the total assessments by the total selling prices. The ratio of total assessments on those houses to total selling prices gives you what's called an "assessment-sales ratio." Let's say the sales add up to $1 million and the assessments to $300,000. That's an assessment-sales ratio of 30 percent. If your assessment is more than 30 percent of your house's current full cash value, you have a strong argument in pressing your appeal.

The considerable research outlined above may not be necessary in certain states. The table on pages 122-125 indicates those states that annually compute the assessment-sales ratio for each taxing jurisdiction. These state-computed ratios should be available from the local assessor's office or from the state property-taxation agency, usually called the Board of Equalization.

But even in those states, there may still be reason to research your own assessment-sales ratio. Because of the inevitable gap between the time the data are gathered and the time they are published, the information is always a little out of date. Some local appeals boards may not accept the state's assessment-sales ratio as accurate evidence in an appeal. (One state where the official ratio should carry weight is New York. A court ruling in 1975 established that the state-computed ratio, called the *equalization rate* in New York, is sufficient evidence about local rates on which to base an appeal.)

A second difficulty is that the state-computed ratio may include in its statistics not only homes but commercial and industrial properties. If you were assessed unfairly in relation to houses, but not in relation to all real estate, the official ratio may not reveal the inequity and may actually work against you, if cited by the assessor.

The assessment on your house is higher than on similar houses in your neighborhood. If you don't have the time, patience, or contacts needed to research an assessment-sales ratio based on a large number of houses, you might simply find out (from the assessment rolls) the assessment on houses in your neighborhood you judge to be close in value to your own. If you find that your assessment is higher, you can appeal it. You would have especially good grounds for appeal if you lived in a development and were comparing your house with houses obviously similar to yours. In this case it is wise to bring to the appeals board photos of the houses you are comparing and, if possible, a typed list of the features of each.

Appeals on the basis of overassessment or unfair assessment are even more powerful if it is also true that:

The appraiser erred when judging the value of your house. Appraisers can make mistakes in recording the features of a house. (It's not unheard of for an appraisal to be made by someone who has driven by a house and not gone inside.) Property records used in appraising a house for tax purposes are normally public records that the assessor should allow you to examine. Ask to inspect these records.

Check to be sure the recorded dimensions of both the house and land are correct. If the basement and attic aren't finished, for example, or if there are room heaters instead of central heating, be certain the records say so. If the front of the house is brick, but the rest is sided with another material, be sure the house isn't described as all brick. Sometimes the volume of the house will be computed in cubic feet and an assessment will be based partially on this figure; do your own measurements and computations to check the figures on the appraisal. Check also to see if the appraiser considered defects that would tend to reduce a house's value. A defect can be anything you don't plan to fix soon. The house might have settled, for instance, as attested to by cracks in the walls. The thousands of dollars it would take to shore up the foundation is a persuasive reason for the assessment to be reduced. If your roof has a fifteen-year life, would cost $2,000 to replace, and is already twelve years old, point this out. A consistently wet basement, a termite infestation, even a rundown backyard are examples of other defects.

How to Present Your Appeal

If you decide that your assessment is too high and you can back up your judgment with evidence, turn to the table on pages 122-125. Listed there next to each state are the name of the assessment appeals agency (or agencies) in that .state's taxing jurisdiction and the dates on which it hears appeals. But before you appeal formally, try to talk with the assessor informally. If you have a reasonable case, many assessors will be happy to avoid the nuisance of defending an appeal by negotiating informally, perhaps reaching a compromise settlement. The assessor will be especially likely to negotiate if you've found an obvious mistake on your property record forms. Even if your appeal will be made on the ground of assessment inequity, the assessor might be willing to discuss the problem.

Learn about deadlines and forms well in advance of any formal appeal. Normally, appeals are heard during only one period in the year, and you can appeal an assessment only for the current year's property taxes. So if you miss that chance to appeal, you miss the chance to reduce the tax burden for a full year. Suppose, for example, the assessment on your house hasn't changed in the last four years. You can still appeal the assessment, asking for a reduction in the present year's property taxes, but you can't ask for a refund to make up for the previous years. Don't wait until your property-tax payment is due; the year's deadline for appeals may have passed by then.

Not all states give you adequate information about your assessment or indicate on the tax bill or the assessment notice the time span within which you can file an appeal.

The filing time for each state is given in the table on pages 122-125. Check dates with the assessor's office (there may be local variations), ask about the necessary forms, and get any instruction booklets that may be available.

Sit in on an appeals hearing to see what it's like. You may get some valuable help listening to other people's grounds for appeal and seeing how the board reacts. Some boards, for instance, might accept the argument that a similar house on your block is assessed at far less than yours; others might dismiss it with the comment that the assessment on the other house should be raised rather than yours lowered. Some boards might accept your research into assessment-sales ratios; others might demand proof that every sales price cited represents market value rather than unusually low price accepted by a seller in a hurry. The assessor and the appeals board may bring up technical points you don't understand. Take notes at the hearings and try to find out about anything you don't understand before your appeal comes up.

But don't let an appeals board or the assessor scare you out of a decision to file an appeal. If you file an appeal in San Francisco, for example, you get a notice informing you that the board determines your proper assessment by "arriving at the fair market value of your property." It warns that the board "may *increase* or lower the assessment" (emphasis ours) and tells you to notify the board if you decide to withdraw your appeal.

Since relatively few houses in California, just as in most of the nation, are assessed at anything close to the actual price they could be sold for, such a message can be quite intimidating. In San Francisco in 1975, 1,381 people, about one-quarter of the total who filed appeals notices, did decide to withdraw their cases before the hearing. Those who withdrew were doubtless unaware that over a seven-year period the appeals board had granted reductions to thousands of homeowners but had only once raised the assessment of anyone who appealed. (On that occasion, the homeowner had appealed for a higher assessment, in the hope that it would help him negotiate a larger mortgage; the appeal was granted.)

Some cities in New York print on their appeals form a warning in red letters that your house will be assessed at full cash value, even though those cities may in reality be assessing houses at an average of 50 percent or less of full cash value. It's not unusual for an assessor or an appeals board member to ask, in effect, "Would you sell your house for the amount it's assessed at? If not, why are you here?" The answer should be: "That's not the issue. The issue is whether my assessment is equitable compared with that of other houses."

At the appeals hearing, don't raise irrelevant issues. Your appeal should concern the validity of your property-tax assessment. An appeals board may well sympathize with circumstances that make it difficult or impossible for you to pay the tax, but the board isn't empowered to deal with such problems.

If you lose your appeal consider going beyond the local appeals board, if possible, in your state. The table on pages 122-125 notes the states with more than one appeals agency. The second or third is usually a city or state agency that will hear an appeal denied by a lower appeals board. Since your case is already researched, there's little reason not to pursue it if you think the local appeals board failed to give you a fair shake.

Local appeals boards can be under considerable political pressure to maintain municipal revenues, perhaps at the expense of the homeowner rather than of commercial real estate interests. Higher boards, though not immune to politics, will at least be one step removed from the pressures of local politics.

The chances of your winning a reduction of your property-tax assessment depends primarily on the strength of the case. If you can show that your assessment is too high in terms of one or more of the appeals grounds we have discussed, you ought to appeal it. But the odds for a successful appeal can vary drastically from area to area. In 1974, roughly 30 percent of those homeowners who appealed in New Rochelle, a city in Westchester County, N.Y., were granted reductions. But in the nearby city of Yonkers the same year, less than 10 percent of appeals were upheld.

Sometimes, the difficulty of appealing may hardly be worth the effort. Norman Taylor, chief of the supply division of the National Bureau of Standards, discovered in 1974 that the assessment on his four-bedroom house in Silver Springs, Md., had jumped 35 percent. Taylor claims there were a number of errors in the appraisal—that the assessor's records show features of the house that do not exist, overstate the size of the house, and understate the depreciation. He also contends his subdivision is overassessed compared with neighboring communities.

Mr. Taylor's attempt to secure a tax refund through the appeals process entered its third year in 1976. He says he has already put in more than twelve hundred hours of time and spent $500 so far. He has consulted Bureau of Census statisticians and tax lawyers to check his methodology, charted sales and assessment records going back to 1968 for six hundred homes in his own and nearby communities. He has submitted a meticulously researched thirty-nine-page argument accompanied by twenty-eight pages of exhibits. But both the original appeals board and the Maryland Tax Court, the second step in the appeals process, turned him down.

WHERE TO APPEAL YOUR ASSESSMENT

Here, state by state, are the basics you must know to appeal your property assessment. Only Delaware, which has a different appeals procedure for each county, is excluded. In some jurisdictions within a state, procedures may vary slightly from that given n the table. Most of it he information has been compiled for CU by the International Association of Assessing Officers; some information comes from interviews with assessors in major cities.

State	Appeals agencies Ⓐ	Time to file Ⓑ	Assessment-Sales ratios Ⓒ
ALABAMA	County Board of Equalization	By 10 days before first Monday in June	No
ALASKA	City or Borough Board of Equalization	By 30 days from assessment notice	Yes
ARIZONA	County Board of Equalization; State Board of Tax Appeals	By 15 days from assessor's appeal decision	Yes
ARKANSAS	County Equalization Board	From first to third Monday in August	Yes
CALIFORNIA	County Assessment Appeals Board or Board of Equalization	Mainly in July and August	Yes
COLORADO	County Board of Equalization; Colorado Board of Assessment Appeals	By second Wednesday in July	No
CONNECTICUT	City Board of Tax Review	In February	No
DISTRICT OF COLUMBIA	Board of Equalization and Review	From first Monday in January to April 15	Yes
FLORIDA	County Board of Tax Adjustment; State Department of Revenue	Usually by July 15	Yes
GEORGIA	County Board of Equalization	By 10 days from assessment notice	Yes
HAWAII	District Board of Review; State Tax Appeal Court	By 25 days from assessment notice	Yes
IDAHO	County Board of Equalization; State Board of Tax Appeals	By second Monday in July and on fourth Monday in November	Yes

State	Appeals Agencies [A]	Time [B]	[C]
ILLINOIS	County Board of Review (or Appeals); State Property Tax Appeal Board	By 20 days from assessment notice	Yes
INDIANA	County Board of Review; State Board of Tax Commissioners	By 30 days from assessment notice	No
IOWA	City or County Board of Review	From April 16 to May 5	Yes
KANSAS	County Board of Equalization; State Board of Tax Appeals	From April 1 to May 15	Yes
KENTUCKY	County Board of Assessment Appeals; Kentucky Board of Tax Appeals	By 5 days after first Monday in June	Yes
LOUISIANA	State Tax Commission; Parish Board of Reviewers	Varies (from August 1 to August 15 in New Orleans)	No
MAINE	County Board of Commissioners or Local Board of Assessment Review	By 1 year from assessment	Yes
MARYLAND	State Property Tax Assessment Appeal Board; Maryland Tax Court	By 30 days from assessment notice	Yes
MASSACHUSETTS	Town or City Board of Assessors; State Appellate Tax Board or County Commissioners	By October 1	Yes
MICHIGAN	Local Board of Review; Michigan Tax Tribunal	By early March	Yes
MINNESOTA	Local Board of Review; County Board of Equalization; State Board of Equalization	By 1 year from assessment notice	Yes
MISSISSIPPI	County Board of Supervisors; State Tax Commission	By first Monday in August	No
MISSOURI	County Board of Equalization; State Tax Commission	By second Monday in July	Yes

[A] Given in order of appeal in each state. After you have tried the appeals agencies, your only recourse is to go to court.

[B] Time given is for the first agency in each state. But check with the assessor or the agency; the time will often vary from one jurisdiction to another.

[C] If your state publishes assessment-sales ratios, they should be admissible in the appeals hearing (see page 118).

123

WHERE TO APPEAL YOUR ASSESSMENT (Cont.)

State	Appeals agencies [A]	Time to file [B]	Assessment-sales ratios [C]
MONTANA	County Tax Appeal Board; State Tax Appeal Board	By third Monday in July	Starting in 1977
NEBRASKA	County Board of Equalization; State Board of Equalization and Assessment	From April 1 to May 1	Yes
NEVADA	County Board of Equalization; State Board of Equalization	From December 1 to January 10	Yes
NEW HAMPSHIRE	State Board of Taxation	By 6 months from receipt of tax bill	Yes
NEW JERSEY	County Board of Taxation; State Division of Tax Appeals	By August 15	Yes
NEW MEXICO	County Valuation Protests Board	By 30 days from property-valuation notice	Yes
NEW YORK	Local Board of Assessment Review	By third Tuesday in June	Yes
NORTH CAROLINA	County Board of Equalization and Review; State Property Tax Commission	By June 30	No
NORTH DAKOTA	Local Taxing District Governing Board; County Board of Commissioners; Special State Tax Appeals Board	By 2 years from assessment	Yes
OHIO	County Board of Revision; State Board of Tax Appeals	By December 20	Yes
OKLAHOMA	County Board of Equalization	By 10 days from notice of increase	Yes
OREGON	County Board of Equalization; Oregon Tax Court (Small Claims Division) or State Department of Revenue; If State Department of Revenue, then Oregon Tax Court	Between first and third Mondays in May	Yes

State	Appeals Agencies	Time	
PENNSYLVANIA	County Board of Assessment Appeals or County Board of Revision	By 30 days from assessment notice	Yes
RHODE ISLAND	Board of Assessment and Review or County Superior Court	By 60 days from publication of tax roll	No
SOUTH CAROLINA	County Board of Equalization; South Carolina Tax Commission; State Tax Board of Review	By 10 days from receipt of assessment	Yes
SOUTH DAKOTA	Local Board of Equalization; County Board of Equalization; State Board of Equalization	From February 1 to May Board meeting	Yes
TENNESSEE	County Board of Equalization; State Board of Equalization	From June 1 to end of session	Yes
TEXAS	County Board of Equalization	By second Monday in May	No
UTAH	County Board of Equalization; State Tax Commission	From May 31 to June 20	Yes
VERMONT	Local Board of Assessors; Local Board of Civil Authority	Varies	Yes
VIRGINIA	City or County Board of Equalization	From January 1 to June 30 (city) or all year (county)	Yes
WASHINGTON	County Board of Equalization; Washington State Board of Tax Appeals	By July 15	Yes
WEST VIRGINIA	County Commission (sitting as County Board of Equalization and Review)	By February 28	Yes
WISCONSIN	Local Board of Review; State Department of Revenue	By 1 week from second Monday in July	Yes
WYOMING	County Board of Equalization; State Board of Equalization	From fourth Monday in May to second Monday in June	No

Ⓐ Given in order of appeal in each state. After you have tried the appeals agencies, your only recourse is to go to court.

Ⓑ Time given is for the first agency in each state. But check with the assessor or the agency; the time will often vary from one jurisdiction to another.

Ⓒ If your state publishes assessment-sales ratios, they should be admissible in the appeals hearing (see page 118).

"I long ago lost any advantage in getting my assessment corrected," Mr. Taylor says. "But it's the principle of the thing. The assessment is wrong, and until it's corrected I'm going to keep pursuing it. My only recourse now is a civil suit and I'll probably do it." He claims that all through the appeals process his major arguments and data were ignored.

His experience, however, is not typical. Neither are the experiences of thousands of homeowners in Cuyahoga County, Ohio, which includes the city of Cleveland. A countywide reappraisal in 1970 by the private appraisal firm of Cole-Layer-Trumble Co. brought a flood of complaints. Cleveland's mayor, Ralph Perk, who was then county auditor, conducted a widespread campaign urging people to appeal—and forty-two thousand did so. Paul Ballou, the county's assessment supervisor, estimates that at least 75 percent of the appeals resulted in reductions, many of them, he says, "for the sake of expediency, to save the time of processing complaints."

Appealing an assessment takes time, persistence, and a certain amount of nerve. Those short of one or another of those characteristics might consider joining with a group of neighbors to take joint action. An appeal through a neighborhood association has several advantages. Members of a group might be able to chip in for legal advice, and they could divide the work of doing assessment-sales studies and other research needed to document a case.

Some groups have won significant victories. In Chicago in 1973, some five hundred taxpayers from two southside neighborhoods worked together to fight their assessments. In one neighborhood, 82 percent of the appellants won reductions averaging 27 percent; in the other, 98 percent received reductions averaging 33 percent.

In Philadelphia in 1974, thirty members of the Southwest

Germantown neighborhood association filed appeals and asked for a joint hearing, claiming their neighborhood was overassessed compared with others. "There was a lot of hostility from the appeals board during the hearing," says one participant, "but when the decision came out, almost everyone got reductions."

Oregon Helps Homeowners

The brochure's cover shows a drawing of a jacked-up house with a dollar sign on it and a puzzled owner looking on. "Property value set too high?" it asks. "Take advantage of your right! Appeal an 'outasight' property value."

The brochure, which outlines the appeals process in simple language, looks like something a public-interest group might put out to spur appeals. Actually, it's issued by the Oregon State Department of Revenue.

Oregon is one of the few states that make a special effort to see that taxes on homeowners are set equitably, that homeowners get full and accurate information with their tax bill, and that avenues of appeal are both easily accessible and fair.

To minimize the inequities that lead to appeals, the state does an assessment-sales ratio for each county. By Oregon law, county assessors must assess property at a minimum of 95 percent of market value, so the state's assessment-sales ratio helps guarantee that the law is enforced.

A change-of-assessment notice in Oregon provides the following information: last year's assessment, divided into land, improvements, and totaled; this year's assessment, broken down the same way; an informal invitation to discuss questions with the county assessor; the assessor's name, address, and phone number; and the address of the county Board of Equalization, for those who want to appeal formally. The bill does not give the property's full market value. But since Oregon is one of the few states where assessments must be set within 5 percent of full market value, the homeowner is able to estimate the full value pretty accurately.

In Oregon, if you think your house is valued too high, the assessor will give you access to a computerized list that makes it relatively easy to find the value placed on comparable houses. (Elsewhere, as we noted, homeowners in search of "comparables" must prevail on real estate agents or bank loan officers for help that may not be forthcoming.)

Should you appeal an assessment to the county Board of Equalization and lose, and if either your land or the house on it is assessed at less than $35,000, you can appeal further to the small claims division of the Oregon Tax Court. The small claims division has one full-time judge who will visit your county to hear the appeal. The appellant gets an instruction sheet describing how to pick comparable houses to prove a case. Ten days before the trial, the appellant and assessor exchange their lists of comparable houses, so each knows what case the other has. The trial is conducted informally; an appellant doesn't need a lawyer. The filing fee is only $1.50.

Needless to say, CU suggests that other states follow Oregon's example.

Where to Get More Help

CU has found in eight states public-interest groups that can either answer questions on the appeals process or provide useful written material. Literature available from these organizations could provide helpful background for anyone thinking of appealing.

Arkansas. Arkansas Community Organization for Reform Now (ACORN) will answer specific questions on the phone. Call (501) 376-7151.

Connecticut. The Connecticut Citizen Action Group offers a booklet entitled "How to Check Your Property Tax Assessment." Send $1 to Box 6465, Hartford, Conn. 06105.

Illinois. Citizens Action has a free booklet "How to Find Out If You're Overassessed and How to Appeal." Call (312) 929-2922.

Maryland. Neighborhoods Uniting will send free material on the state's appeals process. Send a self-addressed, stamped envelope to 3409 Bank Street, Baltimore, Md. 21224. For specific questions, call (301) 732-5005.

Missouri. The Missouri Tax Justice Research Project will send a free booklet entitled "A Homeowner's Guide to Property Tax Appeals." Send a self-addressed, stamped envelope to P.O. Box 8052, St. Louis, Mo. 63156. For specific questions, call (314) 725-9783.

New York. New York Public Interest Research Group will send its booklet "Homeowner's Guide to Property Taxes" for $1. Address requests to 5 Beekman Street, New York, N.Y. 10038. If you have specific questions, call the group's office in Albany at (518) 436-0876.

Ohio. If you have specific questions, call the Ohio Tea Party in Akron. Day: (216) 253-5114. Night: (216) 325-7172.

Pennsylvania. If you have specific questions, call the Pennsylvania Tea Party Taxpayers' Information Project, either in Philadelphia at (215) WA 2-6890 or in Allentown at (215) 439-0997.

A Guide for Renters

The image of a helpless tenant quailing before the landlord has been with us for a long time. The image is not perfectly accurate—but it's still too close for comfort. With a nation-wide shortage of decent housing, landlords can often get away with high rents, sloppy maintenance, and unreasonably restrictive leases.

In recent years, though, tenants have begun to take action to improve their lot. As a result, courts and state legislatures are now more responsive to tenant problems. Tenant activism, including the formation of tenants' associations, parallels other consumer attempts to organize in order to deal more effectively with problems in the purchase of goods and services.

Few consumer commodities are more important than housing, which is in fact a blend of a product and a service. For a great many people in the United States, housing means a rented apartment, and the state of landlord-tenant relations forms a crucial part of the quality of life.

If you decide to rent an apartment, two actions are in order if you want to protect your own interests. One is a careful reading of the lease. The other is a methodical inspection of the apartment. The likelihood of a tenant following those recommendations, however, is lessened somewhat by the nature of the housing marketplace.

HOW TO READ A LEASE

With living units so scarce in many places, landlords are often in the driver's seat. When you're out looking for an apartment, then, it is possible that your tour of the available units will be hurried and casual and you'll have little opportunity for systematic examination. It's possible too that, once you've decided to rent an apartment, you'll find yourself faced with a form lease on a take-it-or-leave-it basis. If you don't wish to sign it, chances are there will be someone who *will* sign. And so, the bargaining power of prospective tenants is not as strong as they might wish.

If you're aware of the problems involved in renting an apartment, you can combat them, at least to some degree. This report will give you some hints on how to read a lease and will provide you with a checklist of things to note when examining an apartment. With knowledge and an organized approach, you may be able to redress, at least in part, the balance of power now stacked against those who rent.

You can use the checklist on page 139 before you move in. And save it as a guide for logging any complaints that may come up during your tenancy. The first part of this report is designed to translate some of the fine print in a lease into plain English—to help you to defend yourself against the more obnoxious provisions commonly found.

Danger Signs in a Lease

Although it's difficult for a tenant to negotiate changes in the lease offered, it's worth a try. Even after you move in, changes in lease terms can sometimes be won from a landlord by an active tenants' association.

The clauses described below are major danger spots on which to concentrate. In quite a few states, many of these clauses have been made illegal by statute or have been ruled unconscionable (and therefore made void) by state courts. However, the official-sounding language of the form lease discourages many tenants from exercising—or even finding out about—their rights. Besides, laws and court precedents vary from state to state. This makes it harder for tenants to become aware of what protections they have.

By all means inform yourself as much as possible about the laws in your own state. Tenants' groups, private attorneys, legal services bureaus, and the state attorney general's office are some possible sources of information. Even if you think an objectionable clause in your lease wouldn't be legally enforceable, you'd be better off having it deleted than relying on the courts. The lower courts, which deal with landlord-tenant disputes, often regard leases as holy writ, to be followed literally. Appeals to higher courts are time-consuming and expensive. And even if you win in court—at whatever level—litigation is at best a nuisance that most people would rather avoid.

To strike a clause, the relevant words should be crossed out, and *both* you and the landlord (or the landlord's authorized agent) should initial the change. This should be done on every copy of the lease that you sign. If you can't accomplish any such changes, the danger-sign list beginning on the next page will give you an idea of what you're getting into. To see whether these danger-sign clauses are included—and most of them usually are—you must read the *entire* document. Lease clauses are typically printed in no logical order, and the most important items are often buried deep within a paragraph.

We present first the meaning of the danger-sign clause in **bold face,** then in *italics* the way the clause might typically read in legal terminology.

You agree that the landlord isn't liable for repairs. There are a variety of ways in which leases state that the tenant must pay rent regardless of whether heat, hot water, and other essential services (such as refrigeration, or elevator service in a high-rise) are supplied and maintained. One formulation of such a clause might be worded as follows: *"This lease and the obligation of Tenant to pay rent hereunder . . . shall in nowise be affected, impaired or excused because Landlord is unable to supply or is delayed in supplying any service or repairs, additions, alterations or decorations."*

This clause sets forth the doctrine of "independent covenants," a hoary legalism still applicable to many aspects of landlord-tenant relations, though not applicable to normal business contracts. The doctrine states that the tenant's obligation ("covenant") to pay rent is separate from the landlord's obligation to provide a habitable dwelling. If the landlord doesn't fulfill his or her part of the bargain, the lease doesn't permit tenants to withhold their rent, as buyers would normally withhold payment for goods or services not delivered. Instead, tenants must sue or pursue some other cumbersome legal remedy.

You pay the landlord's attorney's fees. A typical clause reads: *"The Tenant further agrees to pay all costs, including legal fees and other charges that may accrue in the event distraint proceedings are instituted against the Tenant, or in the event suit for rent or dispossess proceed-*

ings are necessary in order to obtain possession of the premises, or to collect the rent."

A distraint is a seizure of property to collect a debt; it has been made illegal or ruled unconstitutional in many states. A dispossess proceeding is an eviction. Thus, in this common clause you pledge to pay your landlord's legal costs if the landlord tries to seize your property or tries to evict you.

You waive your right to a jury trial. Typical wording: *"It is mutually agreed by and between Landlord and Tenant that the respective parties hereto shall and they hereby do waive trial by jury in any action, proceeding or counterclaim brought by either of the parties hereto against the other on any matters whatsoever arising out of or in any way connected with this lease, the Tenant's use of occupancy of said premises, and/or any claim of injury or damage."*

This clause has the appearance of fairness since the landlord also waives any right to a jury trial. But juries are generally more favorable to tenants than judges are, in the unanimous opinion of tenants' organization leaders interviewed by CU.

You agree to obey rules that may not even have been written yet. A typical formulation: *"The lessee covenants and agrees that all rules and regulations printed upon the back hereof, or hereafter adopted by the lessor and made known to lessee, shall have the same force and effect as covenants of said lease, and the lessee covenants that he, his family and guests will observe all such rules and regulations."*

Rules often include prohibitions against owning pets, practicing musical instruments, playing television sets at certain hours, washing cars, storing baby carriages or bicycles in certain areas, or driving nails into the walls.

Such items as the last are constantly violated by almost all tenants. Who, after all, wants to live in rooms barren of all pictures and decorations? But such picky regulations can be used, subsequently, as a pretext for a landlord to keep tenants' security deposits, or to evict tenants if the landlord takes a dislike to them or wants their quarters for some other purpose (such as rental at a higher rate to a new tenant). Persons active in tenant-organizing sometimes find themselves suddenly in violation of a rule previously ignored by the landlord.

Insist on reading the current rules and regulations before moving into an apartment. In some places they're quite reasonable; in others, not. If you have any bargaining power, try to see that particularly objectionable ones are stricken. As for agreeing to follow any rules promulgated in the future, it's best if you don't and second best if a lease provides some arbitration procedure for the tenant who disagrees with the future rules or if a lease limits the tenant's obligation to follow "reasonable" regulations.

You agree to pay possible extra rent. This clause allows the landlord to raise the rent if operating expenses go up, particularly with respect to water or sewer assessments, real estate taxes, pollution-control equipment, or other capital improvements. Typical wording: *"Tenant agrees, during the term of this lease or any renewal thereof that in the event there shall be an increase in real estate taxes, sewer or water charges above the amount of said taxes, sewer or water charges during the year _____, or an assessment charged by the municipality on the demised premises for any period following the date of commencement of this lease, Tenant shall pay his proportionate share of said tax increase, charge or municipal assessment."*

Some leases that run more than one year may include an automatic increase in the rent for each year after the first, with only the first year's rent prominently indicated at the top of the lease. The increase from year to year may be a specified dollar amount or a fixed percentage, or it may even be geared to the change in the cost of living.

You give the landlord free rein to enter your apartment. Leases vary substantially in the degree to which landlords can barge in unannounced and uninvited. A sample of one of the worst "access-to-premises" clauses: *"Landlord or Landlord's agents have the right to enter the demised premises during reasonable hours, to examine the same, and to show them to prospective purchasers, lessees, mortgagees or insurance carriers of the building, and to make such repairs, alterations, improvements or additions as Landlord may deem necessary or desirable. If Tenant shall not be personally present to open and permit an entry into said premises, at any time, when for any reason an entry therein shall be necessary or permissible hereinunder, Landlord or Landlord's agents may enter the same by a master key, or may forcibly enter the same, without rendering Landlord or Landlord's agents liable therefor."*

Taken literally, that clause means that your landlord can kick your door down to show your apartment to a prospective future tenant while you're not home. In practice, courts have usually ruled in such a way as to restrict a landlord's right of entry to normal business hours and to require that twenty-four hours' notice of entry be given the tenant unless there is a genuine emergency. Courts have also made it clear that the right of access can't be used to harass a tenant. The problem is that you might have to sue to prove that the lease doesn't really mean what it says.

The landlord isn't liable if you're injured or if your property is damaged. Most leases have a list of hazards for which the landlord is not to be held responsible. Typically, the list includes *"falling plaster, steam, gas, electricity, water, rain or snow which may leak from any part of said building,"* and several others.

But form leases differ in a key regard. With some, the landlord is not responsible for injury from the listed hazards *unless* the landlord or the landlord's agents have been negligent. For the tenant, that's the better situation.

The worse situation is that the landlord is not liable even if the damage was caused by the landlord's negligence—and many leases say just that. In some, for example, you agree *"that the lessor shall not be liable for any damage or injury of the lessee."* Or you might agree *"to indemnify and save the lessor harmless from all claims of every kind and nature."*

Such a sweeping excuse from any kind of liability will almost never hold up in court. But if the landlord damages some of your property, you'll probably have to drag him or her into court to recover damages. Were it not for the standard form lease, landlords might be more willing to make reasonable out-of-court settlements. And, of course, the lease can be used to cow tenants who don't know their rights.

You agree no one else will live with you. Most leases prohibit anyone not named on the lease from occupying the apartment. For example: *"Tenant will not use nor permit to be used the said premises nor any part thereof for any purpose other than that of a private dwelling apartment for himself and his immediate family."*

It makes no difference whether the visitor helps you with the rent or not. If, two months after moving into your apartment, you want your widowed aunt to move in with you—too bad. You don't control who lives in your apartment.

Of course, few leases prohibit your having guests overnight. It's long-term stays that may present a problem. If a landlord tries to evict a tenant for having a "subtenant" (unauthorized occupant), one issue a court would look at is how long the guest had stayed. Whether the guest moved in furniture and whether he or she maintained a separate residence would also have some bearing on the case.

Subletting your apartment—that is, permitting someone else to live there while you're away and collecting rent from that person while you continue to pay the landlord—is also flatly prohibited under some leases. Under most leases it can be done, but only if the landlord gives written consent. This restriction has some merit, since it gives landlords some reasonable control over who lives in their buildings. But it's an inconvenience and an added problem for tenants, especially those who travel a great deal. About the best you can hope for here is a phrase in the lease saying the landlord agrees not to withhold consent unreasonably.

Any improvements you build in belong to the landlord. Even though most leases require you to get the landlord's consent before making any alterations, landlords get to have their cake and eat it too. Any improvements the landlord allows you to install become part of the landlord's property, enhancing its value for rental to the next tenant. The clause will read something like this: *"The lessee agrees that no alterations, additions or improvements shall be made in or to the premises without the consent of the lessor in writing, under penalty of damages and forfeiture, and all additions and improvements made by the Tenant shall belong to the lessor."*

This clause is intended to refer to such things as built-in shelves, window seats, wallpaper, and towel racks. The logic is that removal of these items might damage the apartment. Even if the tenant could remove them without damage, however, the lease gives the landlord the right to keep them.

You agree the premises are fine as they are. The windows may be cracked; the refrigerator may be broken; there may be hidden defects in the apartment you won't notice until you've lived there for a short time. But the lease you've signed is likely to say something like: *"The lessee accepts said premises in their present condition."* To buttress this, another clause of the lease will probably say, *"Neither party has made any representation or promises, except as contained herein, or in some further writing signed by the party."* So if the landlord tells you the floors will be sanded and finished for you, get it in writing—before you sign the lease. The Checklist for Renters, which follows, may give you some ideas on what commitments you should seek.

A CHECKLIST FOR RENTERS

You can use the list of questions below to check an apartment before you move in. With some exceptions, you can also use it to log complaints about apartment conditions stemming from a landlord's failure to perform proper services or maintenance. Some questions cannot be answered by simple observation and may require interviewing tenants of other apartments in the building or asking the opinion of someone knowledgeable in building problems (an architect or engineer).

1. What is the rent per month?

2. Is a security deposit required? If so, how much is it and under what conditions is it held?

3. Does the lease say rent can be increased if real estate taxes are raised, sewer or water assessments are hiked, or for any other reason?

4. Do you pay extra (and how much) for utilities, storage space, air-conditioning, parking space, master television antenna connection, use of recreation areas (such as pool or tennis courts), installation of special appliances, late payment of rent, etc.?

5. Read the lease carefully. Mark any provisions that seem especially objectionable to you and try to have them removed from your lease. List any provisions that are not included that you would like to have, such as a sublet clause. Try to have them added.

6. Assess the maintenance services: It there a resident superintendent? Are hours for usual maintenance services restricted? How is emergency service handled?

7. How is refuse disposal handled? Are facilities easily accessible? Are they well kept and clean?

8. Laundry facilities: How many washers and dryers are available? (One washer and dryer for every ten apartments is a good ratio.) Are they in good working order?

9. Building lobby: Is it clean and well-lighted? Does it have a lock or other security provisions? Is there an attendant at the door? If so, for how many hours a day? How are deliveries handled?

10. Entrance and exit: Is there an elevator? If so, is it in good working condition? Are the stairs well-lighted and in sound condition? Are fire exits provided? Is there a fire alarm or other warning system?

11. Hallways: Are they clean and adequately lighted? Are they otherwise in good condition?

12. Are there signs of insects? Of mice or rats?

13. Bathroom(s) : Are the plumbing fixtures in good working order and reasonably clean? Does the hot water supply seem adequate? If the bathroom is tiled, are the tiles sound?

14. Kitchen: Is the sink in good working order, reasonably clean, and provided with drain stoppers? Does the stove seem to be in good working order and reasonably clean? Is the refrigerator in good working order? Does it have a separate-door freezing compartment? If there is a dishwasher, is it in good working order?

15. Air-conditioning: Is the entire building air-condi-

tioned? If not, are there separate units, and are they in good working order?

16. Wiring: Are there enough electrical outlets? (Two or three to a room is the minimum needed for convenience.) Do all the switches and outlets work? Are there enough circuits in the fuse box (or circuit-breaker panel) to handle the electrical equipment you expect to install? (If there is a serious question, get an expert opinion.)

17. Does the heating system seem to be in good working order? Is it providing adequate heat (if it's winter)?

18. Is there a fireplace? If so, are there any signs (such as smoke stains) that it has not worked properly?

19. Windows: Are any broken? Can they be opened and closed easily? Are screens provided? Are there drafts around the window frame? Does the landlord arrange for the outside of the windows (in high-rise buildings) to be cleaned? And, if so, how often?

20. Floors: Are they clean? Are they marred or gouged? Do they have any water stains indicating previous leaks?

21. Ceilings: Are they clean? Is the plaster cracked? Is the paint peeling? Do they have any water stains indicating previous leaks?

22. Walls: Are they clean? Is the plaster cracked? Is the paint peeling? Does the paint run or smear when rubbed with a damp cloth?

23. Telephone: Are phone jacks already installed? Are they in convenient locations?

24. Television: Is the playing of television (or hi-fi) forbidden at certain hours? Is an outside antenna connection provided? Is there a cable-TV connection?

25. Is ventilation adequate? Is there an exhaust fan in the kitchen?

26. Lighting: Are there enough fixtures for adequate light? Are the fixtures in good working order? Does the apart-

ment get reasonably adequate natural light from the windows?

27. Storage space: Is there adequate closet space? Are there enough kitchen and bathroom cabinets? Is there long-term storage space available in the building for your use?

28. Security: Does the entry door have a dead-bolt lock? A security chain? A through-the-door viewer?

29. Soundproofing: Knock on the walls. Do they seem hollow, or solid? Can you hear neighbors upstairs, downstairs, or on either side of you?

30. Outdoor play space (for those who would like it) : Is it provided? If so, are the facilities well maintained?

WHEN THERE'S TROUBLE WITH THE LANDLORD

One day in spring 1974 a young New York woman who makes jewelry for a living left her apartment and didn't return until the next day. On her return, she found sewage had backed up from a drain, ruining some clothes, soaking a radio, and damaging some newly finished jewelry. The tenant claimed she had complained to the landlord in the past about the drain, and he had done nothing. She found the sewage stench made her apartment unlivable, so she moved into her parents' apartment while awaiting repairs. She also stopped paying rent.

The landlord claimed the woman must have left a faucet running while she was away. He claimed she owed *him* money because dripping water had damaged his store downstairs. And, finally, the landlord brought eviction proceedings against the tenant for not paying the rent.

The scene that ensued a few weeks later in New York City's Landlord-Tenant Court was remarkable. The tenant brought in a laundry bag filled with the reeking remnants of the flood. The judge passed the bag around so the attorneys and landlord could smell it. He then found in favor of the tenant, excused her from paying the last two months' rent, and awarded her $84 in property damage.

That victory is symbolic of the new tenant activism. The tactic the tenant used in this case was individual rent withholding. Individual rent withholding, complaints to government bodies, collective rent withholding (rent strikes), tenant organizing, and publicity against the landlord are the means presently available to embattled tenants after reasonableness has been exhausted. We'll examine each of them in detail.

In trying to get your reasonable requests heeded by the landlord or building superintendent, it often helps if you put them in writing and keep a copy. The landlord will then have a tangible reminder of your request and you will have evidence to furnish later if you need to move from cooperation to confrontation. If that boundary is crossed, your next step will often be a complaint to a local government body.

Complaining to Local Government

A visit to city hall should turn up a copy of your municipality's housing code. (In many towns and cities you'll be given a copy.) The housing code (sometimes called the housing maintenance code, residential property maintenance code, or some similar title) is the basic document dealing with the conditions of housing in a community, including rental housing.

On reading it, you may be surprised to learn that you are legally entitled to better conditions than you have in your building. Not that the codes mandate any degree of luxury —far from it. But most municipal codes are rather thorough in setting forth certain basic amenities and services that must be provided, such as hot water, heat, elevator service, light, and ventilation.

New York City's code, for example, specifically requires that between October 1 and May 31 residential apartment buildings be heated to at least 68°F during the daytime (if the temperature outside falls below 55°) and to at least 55° between 10 P.M. and 6 A.M. (if the outside temperature falls below 40°). Plumbing, drainage, and sewage systems must be kept in good working order, which means no leaks or stoppages in toilets or sinks. Appliances installed by the landlord, including stoves, refrigerators, and doorbells, must be kept in good repair. The landlord must provide tenants with individual locked mailboxes, adequate facilities for garbage disposal, and extermination as often as necessary to keep the building free of insects and rodents. The landlord must keep the building clean (except for tenants' apartments) and keep the sidewalk in front of the building free of litter, ice, and snow. And the landlord must paint each apartment at least once every three years, unless the tenant has signed a lease provision saying otherwise. The provisions of New York City's code are roughly representative of code provisions in most large cities throughout the country.

Some problems probably won't be covered by the code. Towns rarely pass ordinances forbidding landlords to allow the aesthetic quality of their buildings to deteriorate—annoying though that is to the tenants. Nor can cutbacks of services, such as reducing the number of weekly garbage collections or reducing the number of maintenance personnel, normally be prohibited under municipal codes. Nonetheless, such basic problems as lack of heat are almost always covered, making the protections spelled out under housing codes very important to tenants.

Municipalities vary widely in how well they enforce their

housing codes. Enforcement all too often ranges from non-existent to poor. Some towns have aggressive housing agencies, however; and in other towns, your own persistence and forcefulness can boost the agency's vigor. While you're at city hall, find out who's in charge of enforcing the housing code. If you have a grievance, consider visiting that agency's office to file a complaint. Before you actually file your complaint, however, there's a very important matter for you to think about: Are you acting alone? If so, you're probably forfeiting one of the strongest resources at your disposal—the other tenants in your building. We'll discuss tenant organizing later. For now, suffice it to say that a complaint filed by a large group of tenants, such as a tenants' association, will carry more force both with the landlord and with the housing agency than your individual complaint will. If conditions in your apartment are unacceptable to you, it's likely that your neighbors feel the same way about conditions in theirs.

In forming a tenants' group in your building, it often helps to consult an established tenants' organization in the area. To find a tenants' group near you, inquire at a local newspaper or legal aid society.

Once you've rounded up other tenants, or discarded that idea as unworkable, your next step is to compile a list of complaints. The list should go into explicit detail: If you think you've been overly specific, you've probably got it about right. (For example, "In master bedroom, on east wall, second pane from top on left side of window is cracked.") CU suggests making four or five copies of the complaint list. Mail one to the housing agency, send one to your landlord, give one to the housing inspector when the inspector comes, keep one for yourself, and give one to the tenants' group, if any.

When you contact whatever agency administers the

housing code, request a visit from a housing inspector to certify the existence of violations. This visit will serve three purposes. First, it will expose your landlord to a court appearance and possible fine if the landlord is found guilty of code violations. The fines themselves are rarely stiff enough to motivate a landlord to improve conditions. But the nuisance and embarrassment of appearing in court might in itself be a motivating factor. (Incidentally, you normally won't have to appear.)

Second, if violations are certified, it puts you on strong legal ground. Should your clash with your landlord develop to the point that your landlord tries to evict you, you will probably be able to claim justifiably that the eviction is in retaliation for your complaint to a government agency. In many places, it would then be up to the landlord to prove that the action was not retaliatory. Retaliatory eviction is against the law in at least twenty-five states. In all events, a record of code violations would certainly make a judge look less favorably upon your landlord, should you and the landlord ever square off in court. Such public records are the best evidence in court proceedings.

The third advantage of a visit from the housing inspector is that if the inspector finds code violations (especially serious ones), you may have the right to withhold your rent payments. This is true only in some states, and only under certain circumstances. (Rent withholding is one of a tenant's strongest weapons. But CU advises tenants to withhold rent *only* after getting advice from a knowledgeable tenants' organization or from an attorney who knows well the rights of tenants—and landlords—in your state.)

At the appointed time meet the inspector, along with as many other tenants as possible who are participating in the complaint action. Give the inspector a copy of the complaint list and a tour of the building, pointing out the items on the list. Do get the inspector's name, badge number (if he or she has one), and a copy of the inspector's report. (Request a copy on the spot; if the inspector can't deliver it, go to city hall later and get one.) The inspection itself is free; there may be a slight charge for the report copy. Many times the inspector will turn up violations you didn't know about, such as inadequate wiring or structural defects.

Care should be taken that nothing in the tenants' quarters themselves could be construed as a housing violation caused by tenants. It's also important to keep evidence of the landlord's violations if they aren't apparent. For example, if there are roaches in the building but they come out mainly at night, some samples should be preserved to show the inspector during the day. In some states, your goal will be to get the inspector to record violations as "serious" or as hazardous to the tenants' health and welfare in order to justify withholding rent. Check with an attorney or a local tenants' organization on this point.

Withholding the Rent

Bringing a complaint against your landlord under a local housing code may have positive results for you. If it does solve your problems, all's well. Many times, however, tenants find that prosecution of code violations is so entangled in red tape as to be of little use—or that landlords simply shrug off the minuscule fines resulting from conviction. If that happens in your case, you need to take stronger action.

One of the strongest weapons the tenant has, when things get down to this stage, is to withhold rent in some way. In this, as in other aspects of landlord-tenant relations, tenants are much stronger when they band together than when they act individually. A rent strike by most of the tenants in a building obviously has a much stronger impact than an individual rent-withholding action. And evictions are very rare in collective rent-withholding actions.

Thirty-one states recognize, either by statute or by judicial decision, the warranty of habitability—an implicit agreement, made by the landlord with the leasing of an apartment, that that apartment is a habitable dwelling.* The major remedy for a breach of the warranty of habitability is some form of rent withholding. So, although some of the cases and statutes in these thirty-one states might not *specifically* give the tenant the right to rent abatement, rent withholding, or rent strike, they do *implicitly* give these rights.

There are two basic kinds of rent-withholding actions. In one, a tenant or group of tenants use some part of the rent money to make repairs to the premises. The amount used is then deducted from the rent paid to the landlord. It's legal to "repair and deduct" in more than twenty states. But most of those states clamp a severe limit on how much money can be used in such an action. In several states the lid is half a month's rent or $100, whichever is greater; in Massachusetts the limit is two month's rent. In New Jersey there is no fixed limit.

The more far-reaching form of rent-withholding is a rent strike, undertaken individually or (better) collectively. The idea is that the tenant or tenants will simply not pay rent until the landlord remedies certain conditions or meets certain demands. It's worth repeating that you should consult an attorney or a knowledgeable tenants' as-

---

*See the table on pages 150-151 for a list of the states that recognize the warranty of habitability. In dealing with judicial decision, be sure to check the jurisdiction of the court making the decision. The court's ruling is binding only on the judge or judges making the decision and on lower courts. With courts of equal jurisdiction and higher courts, the decision may be persuasive but it is not a binding precedent. You can be sure that the precedent is binding, however, only if the decision is made by the state's highest court.

sociation about whether you should withhold rent and how to go about it. Here are some guidelines that may prove useful. Try to get a housing inspector to certify violations in your building. Then send the landlord a written notice by certified mail that you intend to withhold rent if the conditions aren't fixed by a certain date. If that day comes and the landlord hasn't taken substantial steps to meet your demands, you begin to withhold rent.

Sooner or later, your landlord will do one of two things: give in, or try to evict you for nonpayment of rent. If the landlord tries to evict you, you'll get a court hearing at which you raise as a defense to the eviction the landlord's failure to provide a habitable dwelling. Here, of course, an official record that the landlord has violated the housing code is invaluable. (Code violations aren't essential, though. Remember that a smelly bundle was enough to convince one judge that a sewage leak had made an apartment uninhabitable.)

The court may make an immediate determination in favor of the tenant or the landlord. Or it may order the tenant to pay rent to the court while further investigation is made. If the tenant prevails, the court may again order the payment of rent to itself, rather than the landlord, and appoint an administrator to see that the money is spent on repairs. Or the court may order the tenant to pay a reduced amount of rent, reflecting the "diminished market value" of the premises.

Courts almost universally frown on tenants who don't have the owed rent money ready to pay the landlord (or the court) if ordered to do so. From the moment a rent strike starts, then, tenants' money in lieu of rent should be collected (perhaps by the treasurer of the tenants' association) to show a disinterested onlooker that the tenants are really out to improve building conditions, not just to

TENANT PROTECTIONS, STATE BY STATE

Tenant protections change constantly, so although we have tried to give information in this table that is accurate as of September 1976, we cannot guarantee its completeness. We urge tenants to check with tenant groups, housing authorities, legal aid societies, or private attorneys to see what tenant protections exist in their localities. States not included in the table offer none of the listed protections, to CU's knowledge.

	Retaliatory Eviction Prohibited	Security Deposit Law	Tenant May Deduct Repairs from Rent	Warranty of Habitability
ALASKA	Yes	Yes	Yes	Yes*
ARIZONA	Yes	Yes	Yes	Yes*
CALIFORNIA	Yes	Yes	Yes	Yes*
COLORADO	No	Yes	Yes	No
CONNECTICUT	Yes	Yes	No	Yes
DELAWARE	Yes	Yes	Yes	Yes*
DISTRICT OF COLUMBIA	Yes	Yes	No	Yes
FLORIDA	Yes Ⓐ	Yes	No	Yes*
GEORGIA	No	Yes	Yes	Yes*
HAWAII	Yes	Yes	Yes	Yes*
ILLINOIS	Yes	Yes	Yes	Yes
IOWA	No	Yes	No	Yes
KANSAS	Yes	Yes	No	Yes
KENTUCKY Ⓑ	Yes	Yes	Yes	Yes*
LOUISIANA	No	Yes	Yes	No
MAINE	Yes	No	No	Yes*

*By statute.
Ⓐ Tenant protected not by state law but by opinion of attorney general.
Ⓑ Law applies only to Lexington and Louisville.

150

State			
MARYLAND	Yes	Ⓒ	Yes*
MASSACHUSETTS	Yes	Yes	Yes*
MICHIGAN	Yes	Yes	Yes*
MINNESOTA	Yes	No	Yes*
MISSOURI	No	No	Yes
MONTANA	No	Yes	No
NEBRASKA	Yes	Yes Ⓓ	Yes*
NEW HAMPSHIRE	Yes	No	Yes
NEW JERSEY	Yes	Yes	Yes
NEW MEXICO	Yes	No	Yes*
NEW YORK	Yes	No	Yes*
NORTH DAKOTA	No	Yes	No
OHIO	Yes	No	Yes*
OKLAHOMA	No	Yes	No
OREGON	Yes	Yes	Yes*
PENNSYLVANIA	Yes	No	Yes
RHODE ISLAND	Yes	No	No
SOUTH DAKOTA	No	No	No
TENNESSEE	Yes Ⓔ	Yes Ⓔ	Yes*
TEXAS	No	No	No
VIRGINIA	Yes	Yes	Yes*
WASHINGTON	Yes Ⓕ	Yes Ⓖ	Yes*
WISCONSIN	Yes	No	Yes

*By statute.

Ⓒ Law varies from county to county.
Ⓓ Limited to utilities and essential services.
Ⓔ Limited to dwellings in counties having a population of more than 200,000.
Ⓕ Limited to buildings with more than ten apartment units.
Ⓖ Limited to toilet facilities.

151

save money. The collected money can then be deposited in an escrow account under the name of the tenants' association. Or the individual tenants can get money orders made out to themselves. The money orders should be kept in escrow in a safe deposit box at a bank whose location is not revealed to outside parties. This way no one but the tenant has access to the money. Here again advice from a lawyer or tenants' association should be sought; these methods of handling the money may very well demonstrate the tenants' good faith but they are not legally sanctioned.

If a court suggests that the escrow money be entrusted to it, many tenant leaders believe that the tenants should bow to the court's suggestion. Other tenant leaders fear the tendency of courts in their area to be prolandlord, or to let the landlord off after an assurance that repairs will be done or have been done. Tenants often feel their landlord will stop bargaining with them once they have lost the leverage of having the rent money in escrow. This fear can have some validity. CU would advise tenants to visit the court that handles landlord-tenant problems in their home area to form an opinion about the general leanings of the judge or judges. Then they will have a better idea about what strategy to pursue.

Getting Organized

Much of what we've said so far has taken for granted the formation of a tenants' organization or association in your building. Tenants do accomplish much more if they're united than if they try to confront a landlord individually.

How does one go about organizing a tenants' association in a building? Consulting an established tenants' organization in the area is usually a good idea. (In fact, affiliating your building's association with a citywide tenant group is often wise, since it plugs your smaller unit into a source of expertise and tends to give the newly formed unit a stature it otherwise might not have.)

There are certain basic steps to follow in getting organized. Begin by announcing a meeting of tenants to discuss common problems. It's best to hold the meeting just when a breakdown of building services has taken place or when the landlord has just taken some action that gives tenants a common rallying point. A mimeographed notice of the meeting should be put under every tenant's door and posted in public areas, such as the lobby and the elevator. But first those organizing the group should lay the groundwork by visiting as many tenants as possible, personally inviting them to come to the meeting. The approach should be low-keyed; tenants, like most people, tend to be cautious about joining groups or undertaking new ventures.

The first meeting should be a get-acquainted session and a forum for airing grievances. Often, tenants are surprised to discover how many of them have common problems. Tenants should be urged to write down their specific grievances and bring them to a second meeting (and that date should be set before the meeting breaks up). The names, addresses, and phone numbers of those present should be taken down, and a mimeographed list should be distributed at the next meeting. All meetings should be held in the building—in either a public area or an apartment.

At either the first or second meeting, officers should be elected. As a minimum, there should be a president, vice-president, and treasurer. If it's desired, these offices can be rotated frequently, for the sake of keeping participation at a maximum. But it's important to pin down responsibility, lest everyone's business become no one's business. One person might be assigned to write a letter to the landlord, another to deal with local government, a third to seek newspaper, radio, and television coverage of their problem, a fourth to get in touch with other tenants' organizations, and so on.

At the second meeting, tenants' individual grievance lists should be fused into a master list. Priorities should be set for bargaining with the landlord. Grievances might be divided into those common to the entire building and those pertaining to individual apartments. But it should be made clear that the group will fight for the resolution of both. The master list should be sent to the landlord, along with a notice that a tenants' association has been formed. (Both for legal purposes and for morale, the association should have a name, even if it's only Tenants' Association of 111 Smith Street.) If tenants fear harassment, note that the landlord need not be told how many people have joined the association or who they are. The association should constantly try to expand its membership and should keep its doors open for late joiners.

The next step to be taken will vary, depending on the group's evaluation of the landlord. The standard approach would be to ask for a meeting with the landlord to discuss grievances. The association would make it clear that the landlord must meet with it by a fixed date and begin correcting the conditions in question by another fixed date. In some cases, this alone will pressure the landlord enough to achieve real changes. In others, where the meeting with the landlord bears no fruit, the association would proceed to inform the landlord that unless conditions are improved by a certain date, a rent strike will begin.

Publicity as a Weapon

The standard approach isn't always the best one, however. Landlords who derive a very small portion of their revenue from rental income wouldn't be very vulnerable to a rent strike. They might be quite vulnerable, however, to publicity. Some people may take the view that publicity tactics are tantamount to harassment. On reflection, however, one may well conclude that a landlord's failure to provide decent housing to tenants, or to obey the housing code, is not a private matter.

Reports in the local news media can be embarrassing, especially to a landlord of some prominence. Picketing can sometimes be effective, especially if it's done imaginatively. Tenants of a building in New York City drew heavy media attention when they picketed outside Belmont Park Race Track with a dancing horse. A horse owned by the landlord was entered that day in the Belmont Stakes. (In case you think united tenant action is mainly for poor people, it's worth noting that these tenants lived in a building with apartment rents ranging up to $2,100 per month. One member of the tenants' association was a United Nations ambassador; another was a prominent publisher.)

The Belmont pickets had to do a little research about their landlord to uncover the financial interest in race horses. You, too, should do some research to find out what strategy will work best against your landlord. Newspaper libraries, tax records, and the county registry of deeds are some likely sources of information. Talking with tenants at other buildings your landlord owns can help. (Indeed, one of the most effective tactics is for tenants at more than one building to join together.) For detailed information about how to do research on your landlord's property holdings, you can consult *People Before Property*, published by Urban Planning Aid, Inc., 639 Massachusetts Avenue, Cambridge, Mass. 02139.

Getting Back Your Deposit

Up to now, we've been discussing how you can strive for good conditions in your apartment while you're living there. But there may come a time when you want to leave. This presents a fresh problem: how to get the prompt return of your security deposit.

The deposit, usually ranging from one month's to two months' rent, is given to the landlord before you move in. In theory, it's supposed to "secure" your compliance with all the terms of the lease. In practice, it's money the landlord can use to square the account if you default on a rent payment or damage the apartment. One trouble is that "damage" can be a subjective judgment, discernible to your landlord, for example, but not to you. Another problem is delay. In many places there's nothing to tell the landlord how promptly the deposit must be returned to you. Once a tenant has moved out of the area, some landlords' memories seem to become laggard.

To help tenants who face such problems, some thirty-two states have passed legislation affecting security deposits. Usually, the legislation aims at limiting the maximum size of the deposit or requiring the landlord to pay it back after a certain amount of time has elapsed from the termination of the tenancy. At least twelve states require that the landlord pay the tenant interest on the deposit. Such laws are helpful, certainly. And if you're staying in the area, small claims courts can also be a big help.

Many tenants take the law into their own hands by declining to pay the last month's rent. Either implicitly or explicitly, they tell the landlord to "take it out of the security deposit." The point behind the maneuver is that if the landlord wants more money, he or she must sue you, rather than the other way around. Risks are fairly minimal; by the time the landlord gets you into court, there will be at most a few days remaining in your tenancy and a judge is highly unlikely to evict you. But note this well: The tactic is illegal almost everywhere. (It can be legal in Washington, D.C., and New Jersey, *if* the landlord has failed to comply with applicable laws governing the use of security deposits.)

To pursue the return of your security deposit through legal means, some preparation would be useful. It would help to have photographs that show the condition of the apartment when you moved in and when you moved out, to establish that you didn't damage the apartment. The testimony of an objective third party could also be helpful. And it's a good idea when you first move into an apartment to send your landlord a list of existing defects by certified mail (return receipt requested). That list, besides providing an agenda for service, will serve as proof later if your landlord should keep your security deposit on the grounds that you damaged the apartment.

TENANT PROTECTION: PATHS TO REFORM

So far we have provided tenants with self-help information. In many places, however, tenants need more: They need reform of the outmoded laws that give the landlords unreasonable power over their tenants.

No state flatly requires that all tenants be given leases. In the absence of a lease—or of effective rent control—the landlord can pile one rent increase on top of another. When there *is* a lease, it usually gives the landlord all kinds of protection, and the tenant none, as noted earlier. And when the lease runs out, the landlord can raise the rent as high as the nation's chronic housing shortage will sustain. That's pretty high. Moreover, nothing in the typical lease requires a landlord to perform even the most desultory maintenance and repair.

What's a tenant to do? We have discussed some of the available remedies: organizing tenants in the building, complaining to local government, withholding rent. Such remedies can be effective. But they're also arduous for the tenants. And in a state with little on the books in the way of tenant protection, a tenant may feel reluctant to get publicly involved, fearing eviction by the landlord. Tenant leaders interviewed by CU all agreed that determined tenants could successfully resist eviction. But many persons are unwilling to become test cases or front-line warriors in the battle for tenant rights. "Why should I have to police the conditions in my apartment building?" they ask. "Why should I have to withhold rent and be taken into court? Why doesn't the government do something?"

In some places, the government has. The state of New Jersey has done the most. Nearly half of the New Jersey residents are tenants, many of them members of the New Jersey Tenants Organization. That group has pushed a series of protenant measures through the state legislature and supported them in the courts. The first was a law prohibiting retaliatory eviction: No landlord may evict a tenant or refuse to renew a lease because the tenant made a complaint about a housing or safety violation or joined a tenants' association. With that basic protection ensured, tenants could go on to fight for other rights. Among those won for New Jersey tenants were:

■ Evictions are legal only if through a court order.

■ Selling a tenant's property to collect rent due (known as distraint) is illegal.

■ Tenants in a building with dangerous conditions can petition for a court-appointed receiver to collect rents and use them to make repairs.

■ Interest must be paid on tenants' security deposits, and deposits cannot exceed one and a half months' rent. A landlord who unjustifiably keeps a deposit is liable for double damages.

■Municipalities can enact rent control under their general police powers. Since 1973, when that provision was upheld by the New Jersey Supreme Court, some ninety towns and cities have done so.

■ Tenants can make repairs and deduct the cost from rent if the repairs are necessary to make the apartment livable and habitable.

■ A town can, by ordinance, require landlords to put down their own security deposits with the town. The money may be used by the town to make emergency repairs in the landlord's building. The New Jersey Superior Court has upheld such an ordinance passed by the town of Ridgefield.

■ A tenant can be evicted only if, "after written notice to cease," the tenant continues certain forms of undesirable conduct. Those, enumerated in a law passed in 1974, include nonpayment of rent, repeated violations of the lease or rules and regulations, and creation of disturbances.

Such tenant-protection measures have put New Jersey in the forefront of the tenants' rights movement. The measures could hardly have been achieved without the activism of tenants' organizations. Indeed, many tenants in the state now enjoy better conditions without having been activists themselves.

The Uniform Act

The reforms in New Jersey were achieved piecemeal, as were reforms enacted in other states until the early 1970s. Since then attention has increasingly centered on the Uniform Residential Landlord and Tenant Act (URLTA), drafted by the National Conference of Commissioners on Uniform State Laws, recommended by the conference for enactment in all of the states, and adopted thus far by at least six states (see page 162)—not including New Jersey, whose tenant-protection laws are already stronger than URLTA.

One of the most important things URLTA does is to forbid the separation of a tenant's obligation to pay rent and a landlord's obligation to maintain the property. It is this separation (known as the doctrine of independent covenants) that makes the typical lease so unfair to tenants. The landlord's obligations, spelled out in Section 2.104 of URLTA, include (1) complying with all local or state housing codes; (2) keeping the premises in "a fit and habitable condition"; (3) keeping all common areas of the building in "a clean and safe condition"; (4) maintaining "in good and safe working order" all electrical, plumbing, sanitary, heating, ventilating, and air-conditioning systems the building may have, as well as the elevator, if there is one; (5) providing enough facilities for waste disposal; and (6) supplying hot water year round and heat in the cold seasons. If a landlord doesn't comply with those obligations, a tenant can legally cite that noncompliance as reason for withholding rent.

Prohibited under URLTA are some of the restrictive lease clauses discussed at the beginning of this report. A rental agreement may not provide that the tenant agree to pay the landlord's attorney's fees or waive any of the tenant's rights and remedies under URLTA. Nor can a lease include a clause excusing the landlord from any liability.

Security deposits are limited to one month's rent under URLTA, and the landlord is required to return the deposit within two weeks after the end of the tenancy, unless the tenant has caused damage or defaulted on rent. Landlords are required to disclose their names and addresses in writing to tenants, as well as the names and addresses of any persons authorized to manage the premises.

The tenant has obligations, too. These include complying with local housing codes, keeping the apartment clean and safe, not disturbing the neighbors, and obeying reasonable rules and regulations. Rules are considered reasonable only if they apply to all tenants in a fair manner. Thus, a tenant who organizes a tenants' association or otherwise offends the landlord can't be evicted for owning a dog if several other tenants in the building own dogs. If a rule is adopted after the tenant has already signed a lease, and the rule works a substantial modification of that lease, then the rule can't be enforced unless the tenant consents to it in writing.

If a landlord fails to make needed repairs, URLTA allows the tenant to serve the landlord with written notice of the tenant's intention to make repairs at the landlord's expense. If the repairs aren't made within fourteen days, the tenant can then make the repairs and deduct up to $100 or half a month's rent (whichever is greater) from the next rent check to the landlord.

When a landlord has failed to fulfill the obligations mentioned earlier, the tenant can withhold rent altogether and use the landlord's failure as a legal defense against eviction. In court, if the tenant is upheld, the judge will normally order a reduced amount of rent. The tenant can seek a court injunction to make the landlord fulfill obligations under URLTA. (Tenants who follow this last route can also sue to recover damages and attorney's fees.) Or the tenant can simply move out, upon giving proper notice, and be relieved of any further obligations under the lease.

The tenant has recourse to some stiffer penalties if a landlord willfully diminishes services as a harassment tactic or if a landlord illegally removes or excludes the tenant from the premises. In that case, the tenant is entitled to get back the apartment plus a penalty of three months' rent (or the actual damages sustained, whichever is greater). And URLTA includes a prohibition on "retaliatory conduct." If a landlord threatens an eviction because a tenant has complained to a governmental agency about a housing violation or has joined a tenants' association, the tenant is entitled to the three months' rent penalty. The same applies if the landlord raises the rent or decreases the services as an act of retaliation. Evidence that a complaint was made to a government agency within a year of the landlord's action creates a legal presumption that the landlord's conduct was retaliatory. It would then be up to the landlord to prove otherwise.

Six states that have adopted URLTA are Alaska, Arizona, Delaware, Nebraska, New Mexico, and Oregon. Some states that pass the act modify it a bit: Oregon deleted and Alaska weakened the provision allowing tenants to make repairs and deduct the cost (up to half a month's rent) from the rent due. Florida and Virginia have passed their own versions of the act. Florida's version has a strengthened rent-withholding clause; Virginia's is significantly less protenant than URLTA in many of its provisions, including those pertaining to repair and deduct, security deposits, rent withholding, and retaliatory conduct. Hawaii's landlord-tenant law, passed before the final URLTA wording was approved, differs significantly: There are no rent abatement and rent withholding provisions and tenants' retaliatory-conduct protections are more limited than they would be with URLTA. Washington passed a watered-down law based on ULRTA with many protenant provisions deleted. And Kentucky passed URLTA substantially unchanged, but the state law applies only in Kentucky's two largest cities (Lexington and Louisville). A number of other states are considering URLTA.

In CU's view, URLTA would be a step *backward* in those

few localities that have passed extensive tenant-protection legislation, including Massachusetts, New Jersey, New York, Washington, D.C., and possibly California, Delaware, Illinois, and Pennsylvania. "In New Jersey, URLTA is the backlash proposal," one well-known tenant authority says. "There the landlords want it."

Yet URLTA would be a big step *forward* in most states. "It's a fairly conservative but equitable, middle-of-the-road piece of legislation," says Richard Blumberg, staff attorney of the National Housing and Economic Development Law Project, which provides legal aid for tenant causes. CU does not consider URLTA a panacea. But because URLTA —if properly enforced—would go far toward remedying problems that many tenants face, we urge its adoption by all states that do not already have more extensive tenant-protection measures of their own. URLTA can then be strengthened by other legislation or by amendment.

Some Model Leases

In states with little tenant-protection legislation, one way tenants can try to improve their lot is to try to improve their leases. Even in states where the legal climate is favorable, modification of leases to favor tenants can work a big improvement in living conditions. Because of landlords' preponderance of bargaining power, protenant leases are rare. But they have been achieved in some instances.

The greatest collective bargaining success tenants have won so far is a model lease from the United States Department of Housing and Urban Development (HUD). HUD requires the model lease in all housing projects run with its assistance. (Local housing authorities may use a different lease if it contains provisions establishing "no less than the minimum responsibilities and obligations" of the model lease.)

HUD requires that all tenants in its aided housing projects be given written leases. It suggests, but does not require, that security deposits be limited to one month's rent and that no monetary penalties be assessed for late payment of rent. The lease provides that the tenant will be paid interest on any security deposit and that the deposit is to be used only in case of default on rent or for repairing "intentional or negligent" damages caused by the tenant.

The most far-reaching provision of the HUD lease reads as follows: "If repairs of defects hazardous to life, health, and safety are not made or temporary alternative accommodations offered to the Tenant within seventy-two hours of Tenant's reporting same to Management, and if it was within Management's ability to correct the defect . . . then Tenant's rent shall abate during the entire period of the existence of such defect while he is residing in the unrepaired dwelling."

That's the exact opposite of the typical form lease, which says that rent doesn't abate no matter how long it takes the landlord to make needed repairs.

For Nongovernment Housing

For private housing, CU knows of an excellent model lease prepared by the National Housing and Economic Development Law Project (NHEDLP). For copies, write the Project's office at 2313 Warring Street, Berkeley, Calif. 94704. To be used elsewhere, the lease would require minor adjustments to eliminate local references.

This protenant lease looks like the standard form lease it was designed to replace; it features Gothic lettering at the top and small type below. But nowhere in that type will you find a waiver of the tenant's right to a jury trial or a waiver of the tenant's right to sue the landlord for damages. There is no prohibition against pets, no clause requiring the tenant to pay the landlord's legal expenses, and no blanket prohibition against subletting. (A proposed subletting tenant must be approved by the landlord, but the landlord promises in the lease not to withhold consent unreasonably.)

Equally important are clauses that are *not* included in the standard lease. Protenant leases spell out the landlord's responsibilities and give specific conditions under which rent can be abated (and then resumed).

This model lease is not perfect—it contains tiny type and jargon that requires interpretation by a lawyer—but it does provide a basis for negotiated rental agreements and a starting point for tenants or tenants' groups.

Landlord Security-Deposit Act

In 1972, another tenant-protection measure came on the scene, one that seems to CU to be among the most promising yet. It is the landlord security-deposit act.

The principle is simple. If tenants have to put down a security deposit to ensure that they'll meet their obligations, why shouldn't landlords do the same? The tenant gives a security deposit to the landlord; the landlord gives one to the municipality. The size of the landlord's deposit will depend on the number of rental units in the building. The money is kept in an interest-bearing savings account by the municipality, to be used only for emergency repairs. Deposits are not pooled; each landlord's deposit can be used only for repairs in his or her building.

The value of a landlord security-deposit system is that a town can step in and make emergency repairs without going through cumbersome court procedures (during which the tenants sit shivering with no heat or suffering with no water). If a landlord believes that no emergency existed and the security deposit was unjustly tapped, the use of the security deposit can be appealed to the town's governing body (and to the courts).

In 1972, Ridgefield, N.J., enacted a landlord security-deposit act. Since then, other places in New Jersey, such as Fort Lee and Wayne, have followed suit. Hundreds of other municipalities are considering similar measures. Ridgefield's ordinance is administered by a five-member commission that is made up of the borough's health officer, building inspector, one member of the city council, and two members of the board of health.

The ordinance strictly defines an emergency condition as: (1) lack of adequate ventilation or light; (2) lack of properly functioning sanitary facilities; (3) lack of adequate and healthful water supply; (4) hazardous structural, mechanical, or electrical defects; or (5) failure to provide adequate heat. If the commission finds one of these conditions to exist, it gives notice to the landlord. If the landlord doesn't begin making the necessary repairs within twenty-four hours—or if the repairs aren't reasonably complete within seventy-two hours—then the commission steps in and does the job itself.

Strangely enough, since it was passed in 1972 (and upheld by the New Jersey Superior Court in 1973, after a landlord challenge), the Ridgefield ordinance has never had to be used. But according to the registrar of the borough's board of health, "It seems to act as a deterrent." CU believes such an ordinance would be a valuable weapon for any municipality that wishes to help bring about better living conditions for its tenants. A copy of a model security-deposit ordinance can be obtained from the NHEDLP (address on page 164).

Rent Control

Model leases and landlord-tenant reform laws like URLTA

can help tenants achieve better conditions in their dwellings. What they can't do (except in the rare case of a long-term lease) is control the rents tenants must pay.

Landlords like to blame spiraling rents on increasing costs. There's no doubt that the costs of heating oil, taxes, and financing have gone up sharply in recent years. But rents have been soaring for a long time, sometimes disproportionately to landlords' costs. The simple fact is that there are more people seeking decent housing than can be accommodated by the nation's current housing stock and the annual additions being made to it. When demand exceeds supply, the suppliers can call the tune on price.

Solution to the country's housing crisis, however, is probably a long way off. Meanwhile, tenants must live. So in some localities they have pressed for controls on the rents they may be charged. Where such controls do exist, they usually have taken the form of municipal or county ordinances passed under powers delegated by a state legislature. (New Jersey, as mentioned, is an exception: Courts there have ruled that towns can pass rent control under their own general police powers.) States in which at least certain municipalities are allowed to have rent control include Alaska, Connecticut, Florida, Maine, Maryland, Massachusetts, New Jersey, and New York. (The District of Columbia passed its own rent-control ordinance in August 1974.)

Rent control almost always takes the form of a limit on how much landlords can raise the rent from one lease term to another or from one year to another. Such limits have been based on different formulas in different areas. Some are variable from year to year (using the Consumer Price Index or a landlord's increase in operating costs as a base); others are fixed at a specific annual percentage. Most rent-control statutes allow landlords to apply for extra "hardship" increases under certain circumstances. However, this usually means that landlords have to open their books to prove their case, something few landlords have done.

Rent control, in CU's opinion, is a valuable short-term measure to protect tenants. But it's no long-term solution. Indeed, if continued over too long a time, it might frighten off potential investors in the housing field and cause abandonment or inadequate maintenance of existing structures. It's simply not possible to control price rises in one isolated sector of the economy while other costs (including fuel, materials, labor, and the cost of loans) are allowed to rise.

Rent control copes with some of the symptoms of inflation and lack of housing. That symptomatic treatment may be valuable—even necessary. But at some point the disease itself must be dealt with, through policies providing an adequate supply of housing. Otherwise, rent controls may only aggravate the housing shortage by increasing the demand and lessening the supply. This can result in black-market practices (such as kickbacks for getting an apartment in a building ostensibly under rent control) and can work to the special disadvantage of poor people, who are left with the worst housing or none at all.

When it is used, rent control should be coupled with protection against arbitrary evictions. Otherwise, landlords could evict their tenant population periodically to make room for higher-paying renters.

Recommendations

In CU's view, the first essential step toward landlord-tenant reform is that every tenant who wants a written lease be given one—or, if the tenant prefers, a written month-to-month agreement. Without one, tenants don't know where they stand and sometimes can be subjected to arbitrary and repeated rent increases or to capricious evictions. Delaware requires that a landlord accept a lease proffered by a tenant, unless the landlord offers one of his or her own.

Second, each state that doesn't already have equivalent legislation (or an accumulated body of court decisions establishing tenant rights) should pass URLTA. This will make illegal some of the worst clauses that have marred leases, and it will provide tenants protection against retaliatory eviction, a ceiling on security deposits, a list of obligations the landlord must fulfill, and a legal way to withhold rent if the landlord doesn't fulfill those obligations.

Third, CU recommends that each state passing URLTA strengthen its tenant-protection features by amendment and supplemental legislation. The limit of half a month's rent on the sum a tenant can deduct from rent to make repairs should be raised probably to about two months' rent. State legislation should make it explicit that tenants are permitted to undertake a "repair and deduct" action collectively as well as individually. Where appropriate, the basic reform package should be accompanied by rent control as a short-term measure. And a landlord security-deposit act would be extremely helpful in protecting the rights of tenants.

How to Judge a Dentist

Most Americans are all too familiar with dental disease. Half of American children have at least one decayed tooth by the age of two; by the age of fifteen, the average adolescent has eleven teeth that are decayed, missing, or filled. About one-fifth of the population wears full upper dentures by the age of thirty-five, and about one-half of the population has no natural teeth, upper or lower, by age sixty-five.

The conditions that produce those statistics are largely preventable by regular dental care. But about half of the population does not see a dentist regularly—and according to a 1973 National Health Survey, more than twenty-three million Americans have never visited a dentist.

Dentistry has repercussions beyond the mouth. Symptoms of some dangerous diseases, such as leukemia, are often seen first in the mouth. Syphilis, tuberculosis, and diabetes can also cause telling changes in the mouth. The dentist should be able to recognize the symptoms and help diagnose the disorders. Some diseases travel in the opposite direction, starting in the mouth and then affecting the rest of the body. An infection starting around a single tooth, for example, can lead to bacterial contamination of the blood. If misaligned or loose teeth make proper chewing difficult, poor digestion, poor nutrition, and poor health can result.

A good dentist can help save your teeth *and* contribute to your general state of health. A poor dentist, however, may be as bad as no dentist at all. Later in this report, we'll suggest ways that will help you to distinguish the good from the bad.

Unlike medicine, dentistry is still a profession of the generalist; about nine out of ten dentists are general practitioners. But there has been a growing trend toward specialization over the past fifteen years. Qualification in a specialty requires at least two years of training beyond the four years of professional schooling that lead to either a Doctor of Dental Surgery (DDS) degree or a Doctor of Dental Medicine (DMD) degree. In most instances, specialty qualification also requires practical experience in the specialty.

There are eight specialty areas recognized by the American Dental Association (ADA), including orthodontics (the correction of poorly positioned teeth and of oral defects), pedodontics (children's dentistry), periodontics (treatment of diseases of the supporting tissues of teeth), and endodontics (the treatment of diseases of the inner portion of the tooth—the nerve or pulp). In fourteen states, dentists cannot announce that their practices are limited to a specialty without their having first passed an examination in that specialty given by those states.*

Because of the rapid expansion of knowledge in den-

*Those states are Alaska, Arkansas, Illinois, Kansas, Kentucky, Michigan, Mississippi, Missouri, Nevada, Oklahoma, Oregon, South Carolina, Tennessee, and West Virginia.

tistry, dental education should not end with the DDS or DMD or even with specialty training. It is important for dentists to read current professional literature and to take additional courses to learn about the latest facts, techniques, and instruments. Despite the importance of keeping abreast of new developments in dentistry, only eight states (California, Kansas, Kentucky, Minnesota, New Mexico, North Dakota, Oklahoma, and South Dakota) have continuing education requirements for dental relicensure. (The others relicense dentists automatically on payment of a license fee.) The dental societies of seven other states—Arizona, Colorado, Florida, Louisiana, Nevada, South Carolina, and Washington—as well as the District of Columbia require continuing education as a condition of membership.

Since most dentists work in their own offices in solo practice, there is little or no monitoring done by other practitioners or by hospital committees. State dental associations and many local dental societies have peer review committees to deal with complaints from insurance companies, and some associations have patient mediation committees to handle patient complaints. But they offer no protection for patients before or during treatment, depending mainly on complaints after treatment. And because the judgments are made on one dentist's work by other dentists, there is a built-in potential for bias.

Unbiased judgments of the quality of dental care are needed. According to a 1974 survey, one-half of all dental X-rays submitted to Pennsylvania Blue Shield were unsatisfactory for diagnostic purposes. And improper diagnosis can, of course, lead to improper treatment. The United States Administrators (USA), a firm that evaluates the quality of dental and medical care for insurance companies and self-funded health and welfare trusts, has reviewed thousands of cases.

More than 16 percent of those cases indicated a need for dentists to alter treatment plans or to correct defects in treatment. Most of the changes reduced unnecessary or excessive dental treatment, as judged by USA, but USA also recommended additions to some treatment plans—most often fillings for cavities that had not been diagnosed, and additional diagnostic X-rays to ensure a thorough examination. According to CU's dental consultants, there is a great deal of undertreatment, particularly undertreatment of periodontal (gum) disease. Most denture wearers have lost their teeth because of failure to get adequate periodontal care.

That there's a need for more widespread quality review in dentistry does not mean that most dentists do shoddy work. But in dentistry, as in any other profession, there are the competent and the incompetent, and the ethical and the unethical. Patients themselves may sometimes be forced by economic circumstances to opt for dentistry that's less than good—a cheap fast extraction, for example, rather than a more complex procedure to save an infected tooth. Root canal therapy (cleaning out the pulp-filled canals and filling them permanently with inert material) and periodontal therapy (treatment designed to heal or remove diseased gum tissue) are often slow, unpleasant, and costly. But they are designed to preserve natural teeth and so are usually the best dental alternatives.

Some dentists will do more than others to prevent disease and preserve your teeth. Thus, a patient in search of a dentist should try to identify a prevention-oriented general practitioner. Even if you believe that you have severe orthodontic problems or that your gums need a lot of work, general practitioners are more qualified than specialists to evaluate your overall oral condition. They can perform a broad range of dental services and direct you to a specialist if the condition of your mouth requires complex treatment.

You may consider looking for a pedodontist if you have any children who need a first or new dentist. There are about twelve hundred pedodontists practicing in this country, mainly in medium and large cities. But their services are not necessary for routine dental care. A pedodontist is trained to treat children with behavioral problems, handicapped children, and children with unusual dental problems involving growth and development. If you use a pedodontist as your child's primary dentist, you will be paying a premium for the dentist's specialty training even though your child's dental-care needs may be routine. And your child will eventually outgrow the pedodontist and have to switch over to a general practitioner. (Incidentally, our dental consultants suggest that a child first see a dentist when all the primary or "baby" teeth have come in, generally at two or two and a half years of age, unless a problem arises earlier.)

Ideally, you should start looking for a dentist when you don't need one, so you can take your time and make a reasoned, deliberate decision. There are several ways to obtain the names of promising candidates:

■ If you're moving and already enjoy the services of a general practitioner who meets most of the criteria we'll set forth below, your present dentist might be able to recommend colleagues in your new location.

■ If you already know any orthodontists or periodontists, those specialists might be able to direct you to a good general practitioner. They tend to be prevention-oriented specialists who get referrals from dentists who want to save teeth, not extract them. Also, they are in a position to observe the quality of work done by referring dentists.

■ If there is a hospital or a neighborhood health center in your area that provides dental service, ask the dentist in charge for recommendations for you to explore.

■ If there is a dental school nearby, you could call and ask for the names of faculty members who practice in your community. Some dental schools may be able to provide you with that information. Dentists who have teaching posts are often held in high esteem by their colleagues and are interested in keeping up with advances in dental theory and practice. (To locate the nearest dental school, either check with your local dental society or write to the American Dental Association, 211 E. Chicago Avenue, Chicago, Ill. 60611.)

Don't bother with listings in the Yellow Pages, and use local dental societies only as a last resort. They list dentists but don't evaluate them. Your next step is to make an appointment with one of the recommended general practitioners for a consultation. Explain that you are in the process of selecting a personal or family dentist and want to ask some questions. You may meet with resistance. Dentists and their assistants are not accustomed to being interviewed by prospective patients. But you have a right to information about a dentist's practice before you start using—and paying for—a dentist's services. (A dentist could keep costs to a minimum in a first "shopping visit" by having an auxiliary, rather than the dentist, provide most of the information you seek. Or the dentist could prepare a printed sheet with relevant information about the practice.)

When you visit the dentist's office for the first time, there's a lot you can learn simply by looking around and observing the atmosphere, the people, and the pace of the work going on. There are other aspects of the practice that will remain a mystery until you become a patient, interact with the dentist, and judge how well the dental work suits your needs. But even on that first look-around visit, the dentist or other staff member should be willing to answer your inquiries. If not, that's one sign that you ought to look elsewhere.

In evaluating a dentist, take into account the factors listed below. Some will influence your initial choice of a dentist. Some may make you glad you made that choice. But no matter how careful you are, some may indicate that you've made a mistake and need to start again.

Consider the dentist's location and office hours with special care. The office should be in a convenient location, and the office hours should be compatible with your schedule. Otherwise you may tend to put off necessary maintenance work.

Find out how the dentist provides for care in emergencies. It is the dentist's responsibility to see that emergency care is provided whenever a patient needs it. Some dentists have twenty-four telephone coverage. Some arrange for another dentist to be on emergency call if they are away or unavailable.

Ask about the average wait between the request for an appointment and the date of the appointment. In 1972, the average wait for an appointment with a general practitioner was about two weeks. If you consistently have to wait much longer than that, it may discourage you from seeing the dentist and may delay your treatment.

Take a good look around the office to see how it really works. The office should be clean and neat and the staff personable. Pay particular attention to the flow of patients in the office. If the waiting room is crowded with patients who appear to have settled in for a long wait, it may indicate a lack of organization and proper scheduling.

To provide high-quality care, a dentist should schedule specific appointments of a reasonable length of time—generally at least half an hour. The dentist should stick as closely as possible to that schedule to keep waiting time to a minimum when emergencies don't intervene. And the dentist should tell scheduled patients when an emergency upsets the schedule.

The efficiency of modern dentistry and current pain-control techniques allow dentists to work with a patient for relatively long periods. If they are not doing it—if a patient has to return repeatedly for small bits of work—they are not providing the best possible care. And dentists who hop from chair to chair a lot, trying to do the most work in the least time, are shortchanging their patients. Good dental work requires concentrated attention, not constant motion. **Find out if the dentist makes regular use of auxiliary personnel.** The number of dental auxiliaries—dental hygienists, dental assistants, and laboratory technicians—has increased markedly since 1960; auxiliaries now outnumber dentists themselves. Dentists who don't employ auxiliaries should not automatically be dismissed from consideration. But prospective patients should understand the function of auxiliaries and the advantages and disadvantages of their use.

The dental *hygienist* scales and polishes teeth, takes X-rays, applies fluorides and other preventive agents to teeth, and instructs patients in proper oral hygiene and diet.

The dental *assistant* prepares the patient for treatment, prepares the dental materials, and passes instruments and materials to the dentist. Dentistry in concert—by a dentist and dental assistant—is known as four-handed dentistry.

The dental *laboratory technician* constructs dentures, crowns, bridges, and orthodontic devices. Most technicians work in commercial dental laboratories, but a growing number are employed by private dentists.

If auxiliaries are used effectively, the productivity and

efficiency of a practice can increase enormously. The dentist can devote more time to procedures requiring a higher degree of training and experience. In forty-six states, auxiliaries are permitted to perform some "expanded" functions previously reserved for the dentist, such as taking impressions for study casts and removing sutures. In a few states, specially qualified auxiliaries are permitted to place and carve fillings after the cavity has been prepared by the dentist.

Some patients may prefer a one-to-one relationship with the dentist: They may feel that auxiliaries turn dentistry into an assembly-line process. But a dentist and assistant working in harmony can do more work in less time than a dentist alone. And the team approach can lead to less discomfort for the patient—as the dentist concentrates on performing the dental procedure, the assistant is free to administer to the patient's needs (changing cotton rolls and gauze pads, for example, and using suction apparatus during drilling).

Take note of whether the dentist gets a good medical and dental history. Some medical conditions, such as heart disease, diabetes, and hormonal disorders, may require the dentist to take special precautions. The dentist should find out what medication you are taking and if you have any drug allergies. To learn as much as possible about your dental status, the dentist should try to obtain copies of X-rays and written records from your previous dentist. A dentist who knows how long you've had certain conditions, and how fast they've been progressing, can treat them more effectively.

Consider how thoroughly the dentist examines your teeth and entire oral cavity. You should receive a complete examination when you first see a dentist and at least every three to five years thereafter. (You should have recall checkups at shorter intervals, but they need not be as extensive.)

A thorough examination includes:

- Checking external structures, the jaw joint, facial muscles, and the entire mouth for signs of irritations and tumors.
- A close examination of the teeth for cavities and out-of-place teeth.
- An examination of the gums, including the use of a millimeter probe to measure the depth of periodontal pockets—areas of separation between gum and tooth caused by a build-up of bacteria and calculus (known as tartar).
- Making of molds, or study models, of teeth when required for accurate diagnosis. Molds are generally needed if a patient has teeth missing or a distorted bite but not if a patient has a full complement of teeth in good shape.
- Taking necessary X-rays. It is no longer accepted dental practice to take a complete series of X-rays every six months. According to the ADA, X-rays should be taken only when necessary for proper diagnosis.

There is widespread disagreement among dentists about how often a full series of X-rays ought to be taken. CU's dental consultants suggest that a full series be taken no more often than every three to five years; a survey of decay with two to four X-rays, called "bitewings," may be used in the interim. If your dentist *never* X-rays your teeth, look for another dentist.

To minimize X-ray risks, dentists should use properly shielded equipment, high-speed film, short exposures, and a lead apron for children and all patients in the reproductive age range (and for any other patient who requests one).

Expect a dentist to keep you informed and explain treatment alternatives. Once the examination has been com-

179

pleted and the dentist has had a chance to study its results, the dentist should describe to you the condition of your mouth and what corrections, if any, need to be made. A good dentist will discuss alternative treatments and describe possible benefits and complications of any proposed treatment.

Alternative methods of treatment are more common in dentistry than in medicine. For example, a tooth with a large cavity may be treated by extraction, by root canal therapy followed by a silver filling, by the insertion of a gold inlay, or by the construction of a crown. When there are reasonable alternatives, it is up to the patient to make the final decision.

Get a written estimate of fees before treatment and itemized bills after. At the treatment-planning session, the dentist should also give you a written estimate of how long the proposed treatment will take and what it will cost. Methods of payment should be discussed before treatment begins. For extensive dental work, installment plans are sometimes available. After treatment the dentist should send you an itemized bill. If a tooth has been filled, the bill should indicate how many surfaces of the tooth were involved.

Watch out for overcharging. Such factors as skill, reputation, and experience figure into a dentist's fees. But you may be charged considerably more by one dentist than by an equally competent dentist in the same community, even though the cost of conducting a dental practice is usually not very different from one part of a community to another. To familiarize yourself with fees for some common dental procedures, see the listing of average fees by states on the following pages.

Choose a dentist who is oriented to preventing disease. Before treatment begins, you should be instructed in how to

DENTAL FEES BY STATE

The following table shows the estimated average rates charged by general practitioners for thirteen dental procedures (we have rounded the averages to the nearest dollar). The figures are based on an American Dental Association survey of June 1973, adjusted on the basis of increases in the dental portion of the Consumer Price Index through August 1976. (CU was forced to use 1973 data because the ADA refused to make public the results of its more recent 1975 fee survey.) The 1973 ADA figures have been increased by 24.8 percent—the percentage increase between 1973 and the first eight months of 1976 in the average index of dentists' fees in the Consumer Price Index. Remember that the figures in the table are state averages; dental fees in cities will usually be higher than those in rural areas.

	Initial examination	Complete X-ray series	Cleaning	Silver filling (one surface)	Silver filling (two surface)	Gold inlay (two surface)	Porcelain crown	Gold crown	Root canal therapy (one canal)	Complete upper denture	Standard removable bridge	Permanent bridge (replacing one tooth)	Simple extraction
ALABAMA	$ 6	$24	$12	$11	$15	$84	$125	$115	$84	$195	$208	$342	$11
ALASKA	12	32	26	17	25	107	188	151	112	306	339	441	21
ARIZONA	8	23	15	12	18	89	146	126	98	264	259	359	14
ARKANSAS	6	24	13	11	15	78	121	102	89	184	191	295	10
CALIFORNIA	8	25	17	15	21	97	150	129	105	314	265	371	16
COLORADO	7	26	15	11	18	84	138	120	93	270	247	343	13
CONNECTICUT	8	25	14	11	17	104	171	161	114	303	286	491	15
DELAWARE	8	24	14	11	18	91	189	159	96	290	280	488	13
DISTRICT OF COLUMBIA	12	25	16	13	20	91	173	157	93	310	277	478	15
FLORIDA	11	26	15	12	19	109	159	143	104	263	281	431	14

181

	Initial examination	Complete X-ray series	Cleaning	Silver filling (one surface)	Silver filling (two surface)	Gold inlay (two surface)	Porcelain crown	Gold crown	Root canal therapy (one canal)	Complete upper denture	Standard removable bridge	Permanent bridge (replacing one tooth)	Simple extraction
GEORGIA	$8	$24	$12	$11	$17	$96	$147	$134	$98	$216	$231	$411	$12
HAWAII	8	22	15	10	17	86	162	113	87	279	271	342	15
IDAHO	6	23	14	10	15	72	122	104	77	214	232	300	11
ILLINOIS	7	23	13	11	17	82	137	124	89	282	273	359	13
INDIANA	7	24	12	11	16	91	136	120	87	232	210	355	11
IOWA	6	23	12	10	16	71	132	106	73	227	217	311	11
KANSAS	7	24	12	11	17	81	136	108	87	244	234	318	13
KENTUCKY	6	24	13	10	15	85	131	115	87	203	203	332	11
LOUISIANA	8	28	13	10	16	89	141	126	93	243	230	370	12
MAINE	6	21	11	10	14	85	137	136	77	194	194	421	10
MARYLAND	9	24	14	11	18	99	172	163	102	285	257	486	15
MASSACHUSETTS	9	23	12	10	16	99	162	160	98	256	248	483	12
MICHIGAN	9	24	14	11	18	102	153	145	99	277	277	411	14
MINNESOTA	6	22	13	10	17	74	140	113	79	251	252	322	12
MISSISSIPPI	7	25	13	11	16	82	129	112	90	199	220	335	11
MISSOURI	7	24	14	11	16	85	132	112	82	256	247	328	12
MONTANA	7	25	14	10	16	86	145	119	82	249	256	327	12
NEBRASKA	8	21	12	11	17	66	127	102	76	234	218	279	12

NEVADA	11	22	18	13	18	85	140	126	98	293	297	376	17
NEW HAMPSHIRE	11	25	12	10	16	90	155	150	100	233	223	447	12
NEW JERSEY	9	24	15	11	18	97	178	170	107	299	277	517	15
NEW MEXICO	6	24	14	11	16	97	138	118	100	238	195	309	12
NEW YORK	8	23	14	11	18	102	171	159	101	295	285	492	15
NORTH CAROLINA	8	24	14	13	16	92	145	128	101	195	216	376	12
NORTH DAKOTA	6	22	13	10	15	76	135	115	83	226	255	313	10
OHIO	7	24	13	11	16	89	148	134	99	261	254	404	13
OKLAHOMA	9	24	13	11	17	90	144	115	94	238	240	342	13
OREGON	8	23	15	11	18	81	134	115	85	268	275	334	13
PENNSYLVANIA	9	23	12	10	15	83	152	148	96	239	228	430	12
RHODE ISLAND	10	25	12	11	17	101	164	146	112	252	334	438	13
SOUTH CAROLINA	7	24	12	10	16	88	140	128	99	191	188	385	11
SOUTH DAKOTA	5	21	12	10	16	74	129	107	74	219	217	294	13
TENNESSEE	8	27	12	11	16	87	138	117	99	221	218	344	18
TEXAS	9	25	14	12	18	90	146	119	107	259	257	345	13
UTAH	6	22	13	9	15	75	122	106	75	224	225	311	13
VERMONT	11	22	11	9	15	102	168	153	102	224	213	468	11
VIRGINIA	8	25	13	11	16	88	150	140	94	245	234	420	12
WASHINGTON	8	23	16	11	19	93	138	120	93	266	267	342	13
WEST VIRGINIA	8	23	12	9	15	80	126	115	86	188	192	345	9
WISCONSIN	6	24	13	10	17	87	147	125	93	269	268	359	12
WYOMING	7	24	16	10	17	77	140	111	76	240	238	317	12

prevent dental disease. The dentist or dental hygienist should show you how to use a toothbrush and dental floss properly to remove plaque—a sticky, almost colorless film of bacteria that forms continuously on teeth and that leads to both decay and periodontal disease. The health worker should also discuss diet with you and the use of fluorides for children and decay-prone adults.

Some dentists set aside special areas for plaque-control programs and have personnel specifically assigned to it. Some use posters and magazine articles and even slide shows to stress the importance of prevention.

Other dentists may not have such elaborate programs, but that doesn't mean they won't get as good results. What is important is a dentist's belief that dental disease can and should be prevented and a willingness to make a sustained effort to impart the knowledge of prevention to patients. As part of the preventive philosophy, a dental office should have a well-functioning recall system so that a patient's progress toward oral health can be periodically checked. In most cases, the appropriate interval between checkups is no longer than one year; usually it's less.

Be wary of dentists who think they can provide all dental services. General practitioners can't do everything for all of their patients. If a dentist claims to be able to perform all dental procedures, no matter how complex, that dentist is not the one for you. General practitioners are, however, trained to do the routine tasks of each of the specialties. For example, general practitioners are trained to tilt an individual tooth and to work with simple orthodontic appliances, but for changing jaw relations or moving multiple teeth, an orthodontist should be consulted. A general practitioner can remove a simple third molar (wisdom tooth), but if it's impacted—wedged between the jawbone and another tooth—that's usually a job for an oral surgeon. A general practitioner is qualified to do routine root canal work, particularly of front teeth. But for back teeth—hard-to-reach and multirooted—an endodontist's skills may be required. Those rules are general. A particular general practitioner may be thoroughly grounded in a particular specialty. But a general practitioner can't be thoroughly grounded in every specialty and should be willing to call in a specialist when needed.

Look for a dentist who tries to reduce the pain of dentistry. Local anaesthetics can numb your mouth enough that you can't feel a thing. And the injection itself is no longer very painful because of the development of sharp, disposable needles. Dental work itself has also become less painful with the development of high-speed drills, ultrasonic cleaning to remove calculus, and electrosurgery for removing tissue.

Tolerance for pain differs from person to person. If you want a stronger anaesthetic or a sedative—or if you feel you can bear the procedure without any pain control let your dentist know. Your dentist should be understanding of any fears you may have and try to work them out with you. If you can't bear the pain of dental work and your dentist does nothing to alleviate it, look for another dentist.

Judge a dentist's treatment as best you can. Patients can't judge a dentist's technical skills precisely. Even dentists who are patients are not infallible judges of the treatment they get. But there are ways a patient can distinguish good dentistry from bad dentistry. And there are ways you can tell if you are getting too much dentistry.

A good dentist will make every effort to save your teeth rather than extract them. Before you have a tooth removed, consider seeking an independent opinion from another dentist. It's a good idea to consult an endodontist, a specialist who is devoted to preserving damaged teeth.

A good dentist will have a light touch and will administer relatively painless injections. During prolonged drilling, the dentist will occasionally pause so the patient can relax and rest the jaw joint. During drilling, the drill should be cooled with water spray. Otherwise, the heat generated by its high speeds may cause biological alterations in the tooth surface, and possibly even nerve death.

During the filling or the placement of a crown, it's good practice to keep the area being worked on free of saliva. That can be accomplished either with a rubber dam—a rectangular piece of rubber used to isolate the tooth being treated from the rest of the mouth—or with cotton rolls and a saliva suction device. Once a restoration is completed, dentists who take pride in their work will polish the filling. Polishing takes some extra time, but it makes the filling look and feel better and tends to discourage further decay.

If a filling is contoured properly, it should feel comfortable to the patient and not seem to get in the way. And fillings should not fall out or crack easily. Porcelain and plastic fillings should last, on the average, about five years, and silver fillings at least ten. Crowns and bridges should rarely need replacement in less than ten years. (The life of a restoration generally depends on both the quality of dental care *and* a patient's oral hygiene and biting habits.)

After treament, your mouth should feel comfortable and function well, your bite should feel natural, and your gums should not bleed. A dentist should pay close attention to the condition of your gums, examining them carefully, teaching you how to care for them at home, and treating them when necessary. But in some offices the gums may be a target of overtreatment. Encourage your dentist to try a conservative treatment approach, such as gingival curettage—removal of calculus and infected soft tissue from the gums—and home care, instead of extensive periodontal surgery.

If your dentist believes surgery is necessary, ask for a consultation with a periodontist.

A good dentist will usually proceed directly to a permanent filling when a filling is needed. Question a dentist who fills your teeth with one temporary filling after another. It may mean that the dentist has a high-volume practice and is not willing to spend enough time with you, or it may mean more visits, and thus more money for the dentist. Occasionally, a temporary filling is useful as a vehicle for sedative medication, but it should be replaced by a permanent restoration as soon as possible.

If you feel pain after every dental visit, if you have bleeding gums and your dentist is not treating them, if your bridges frequently work loose, if your prostheses are uncomfortable and you can't chew properly despite repeated visits to your dentist, it may be time to look for another dentist.

You should also watch out for eager-beaver dentists. Does your new dentist seem to find a lot more work to do in your mouth than your old one ever did? Do many of your silver fillings suddenly need replacing by gold inlays? Do many of your own teeth suddenly need to be cut down and capped? (Caps are also called jackets or crowns.) Maybe you *do* need those procedures performed, but the dentist may be trying to maximize income at your expense. If you suspect you're being overtreated, consult another dentist— one not connected with your present dentist in any way. You might consider using the teaching clinic of a dental school to check on your dentist's recommendations.

The rules outlined above apply not only to dentists who practice alone, but also to those who practice together. In group practice, dentists engaged in the same specialty (such as oral surgery, endodontics, or general practice) or dentists in different specialties work together under one roof and share facilities and personnel. Some groups include both dental and medical practitioners, such as internists, gynecologists, pediatricians, and dental general practitioners.

The number of group practices is growing in most parts of the country. On the plus side, dentists in a group can review each other's work and see to it that a substandard dentist does not remain in the group very long. If they all practice one specialty, they can easily cover for each other in emergencies and over vacations. Because the patient's records are on hand, they know the status of the patient's dental health and can apply that knowledge to the current problem. Also, because of the available coverage, dentists can take time off for postgraduate courses and other training programs—training that may improve their dental skills. If the dentists are in different specialties, they can provide patients with a kind of "one-stop shopping," reducing the fragmentation of dental care. (If medical specialties are also represented, the fragmentation of health care as a whole is reduced.) Whatever type of group practice it is, participating dentists represent the totality of all their years of experience and the variety and complexity of dental problems they each have tackled. Patients can only benefit from that depth and range of dental knowledge.

Not every group is good. If incompetent dentists get together, they will not provide competent care. By using our guidelines, you will improve your chances of receiving competent dental work, whether by a solo or group practitioner. But even if a group practice meets all our criteria, it's possible that it may not be personalized enough for you because you may not always be treated by the same dentist.

Although group practice may lead to economies, patients don't seem to benefit from them. According to a 1971 ADA survey of fees charged for five dental services, the average fees of dentists who shared expenses and of dentists in an incorporated practice were with few exceptions higher than the survey average.

You may not be able to afford a private dentist, or you may prefer to try another type of dental service. If you live near a dental school, you might wish to have all your dentistry done by students at its clinic. Fees are generally low, and the work is closely supervised by professors. Because of the built-in review system, the final product is likely to be good. But the final product will probably take a long time to arrive at. Students work slowly, and your treatment may seem to go on and on and on. But if you have the time, you can get good work for relatively little money.

Many state or local health departments offer dental services free or at reduced cost to poor and handicapped people. In addition, such programs as Medicaid, Head Start, and neighborhood health centers sometimes provide free or low-cost dentistry. Check with your nearest health or welfare department to see if you're eligible. Some voluntary organizations also sponsor dental programs.

Evaluating dental care is not an easy job for consumers. The profession does not encourage "shopping around." Choosing a dentist would be a lot easier if there were community directories of dentists, listing relevant facts about their backgrounds and practices. In the September 1974 issue of CONSUMER REPORTS, CU discussed the development of local directories of physicians. The Health Research Group (HRG), a Washington-based public-interest organization, drew up the first such directory, *A Consumer's Directory of Prince George's County (Md.) Doctors*. Groups in other areas have since followed suit.

It's now the dentists' turn. The HRG published a directory of dentists in the District of Columbia in 1975, and public-interest groups in Newport, Ky., and Etna, N.Y., also drew up directories giving information about dentists. If you would like to perform a valuable service for your community, you might consider drawing up a directory of local dentists either through a group you already belong to or by getting together with some interested neighbors. Information about dentists' practices should be readily available to prospective patients, and you can help make it so. For information on how to proceed, write to the HRG at 2000 P Street, N.W., Washington, D.C. 20036.

Role of State Licensure

A dental school graduate can't just hang out a shingle and set up shop. To receive a license to practice, the graduate must first pass a written examination as well as a clinical (performance) examination given by the state in which the graduate expects to practice or by one of the regional boards (see below). The written examination prepared by the National Board of Dental Examiners is accepted by the District of Columbia and all of the states except Alabama and Delaware. (Nineteen states also offer their own written examinations.)

Dentists who later wish to practice in a different state may have to surmount another hurdle. Seventeen states— Alabama, Alaska, Arizona, California, Delaware, Florida, Georgia, Hawaii, Idaho, Louisiana, Nevada, New Mexico, North Carolina, Oregon, South Carolina, Texas, and Utah —refuse to recognize a license granted by another state and thus make it difficult for established dentists to begin a new practice within their borders. The remaining states and the District of Columbia are more hospitable—to some dentists, from certain states, under specified conditions.

In many states, increasing numbers of out-of-state dentists find their paths to licensure neither totally blocked nor wholly obstacle-free. For those dentists who take part in one of three regional testing programs—which cover thirty states in all—it may be relatively simple to establish a practice in another state, so long as the new state falls within the same testing region. Reciprocity does not as yet extend beyond the states in each test grouping—a limiting factor particularly for dentists in the new four-state Southern Regional Testing Agency, which began operation in 1976.

Because regional testing was unknown before the 1960s, that route to reciprocity is virtually closed to older dentists who wish to practice in another state but who do not want to subject themselves to regional testing. Such dentists might consider moving to one of the twenty-three states that rely on "licensure by credentials." In those states (some also participate in regional testing), dentists who have practiced a minimum of five years and who meet certain other requirements may be deemed to have suitable credentials for licensure. Or dentists who live in one of the handful of states still participating in reciprocal licensure arrangements with just a single other state may move freely to that one other state where by pre-existing agreements their licenses will be recognized.

Even states with regional testing, licensure by credentials, or reciprocity programs still require some additional evidence of competence from out-of-state applicants. One of the more frequent requirements is demonstrated knowledge of the state's dental laws. No state licensing boards rubber-stamp licenses granted by other states.

When a licensure system based on state board examinations began to evolve in the mid-1800s, there was a good reason for it—to protect the public from dentists trained by unqualified, unsupervised schools. But other quality controls have since developed, such as the accreditation of dental schools by the Commission on Accreditation of the ADA and also the written national examination, which is currently accepted by most of the states.

Currently, the state licensure system is a hotly debated subject among dentists. Some contend that the examinations are necessary to maintain high quality in the profession. Others accuse state boards of using the examinations to protect the economic interests of dentists already practicing in those states rather than to test competency.

Just how does restricting the flow of dentists from state to state affect consumers? Not for the better, it would seem. Fewer dentists are available in the so-called "Iron Curtain" states—those that don't recognize licenses granted by other states—than elsewhere. The Department of Health, Education, and Welfare has declared more than twenty areas in Florida to be areas of critical dental shortage. Yet Florida does not recognize dental licenses from any other state, and its state board turned down almost one-fifth of its license applications in 1975. Mississippi has only one dentist for every thirty-four hundred people; until July 1976, when licensure by credentials became effective, Mississippi did not accept dental licenses from any state except Tennessee. Connecticut, in contrast, a state that does accept the licenses of the fourteen other states in its regional testing program, has one dentist for every fourteen hundred people.

In a 1972 poll by the ADA, 70 percent of those responding favored nationwide reciprocity—meaning that a licensed dentist in one state may apply for and receive a license in any other state without taking an additional examination or fulfilling any other requirement. Nationwide reciprocity might help relieve shortages resulting from maldistribution of dentists. But it's feasible only if state boards base their clinical examinations on uniform standards. All states could then recognize, with complete confidence, the licenses granted by other states.

When introduced in 1975, the health manpower bill (signed into law in October 1976) contained useful provisions affecting dental licensure. Those provisions—dropped in the final version of the bill—included setting federal minimum standards for state licensing boards. The license of a practicing dentist would have been recognized in states where national standards were in effect. If a state's licensure program exceeded national standards, however, an out-of-state dentist would have had to comply with those requirements (except any length-of-residence requirement).

How to Find a Doctor for Yourself

One hears a lot these days about the "disappearance" of the old-time family doctor. But if we define a family doctor as one who acts as an all-around medical adviser for the family or individual, treats many ailments personally, and calls in help for a difficult problem, family doctors really haven't disappeared at all. The confusion arises because people continue to identify personal or family doctors with general practitioners.

Many people still limit themselves to general practitioners when they seek personal physicians. To understand why this sometimes brings disappointment, we need to review what has happened in the medical profession in recent decades.

Before World War II roughly 65 percent of all practicing physicians were general practitioners; today about 36 percent are, according to recent American Medical Association

This report was based on two chapters in CU's book *The Medicine Show.*

figures. One reason for the decline is a change in the structure of American medicine, which began with the formation of medical specialty boards. The first one was established in ophthalmology in 1917. Today there are twenty-two such groups, all members of the American Board of Medical Specialties. Each of these boards is responsible for the establishment of training requirements, other qualifications, and the administration of certifying examinations in a particular specialty area. A physician who passes the American Board examination within a specialty area becomes *board-certified* and is known as a diplomate of that board. Many physicians who are *board-eligible* by virtue of their training do not choose to take the certification examinations.

In many of the board specialties, a doctor may also be a member of a "college," an honorary body whose main concern is continuing medical education within the specialty. Once certain qualifications have been met, the physician may be elected to fellowship in the college. Such organizations include, for example, the American College of Obstetrics and Gynecology, the American Academy of Pediatrics, the American College of Physicians, and the American College of Surgeons. Thus such initials as FACOG, FAAP, FACP, and FACS after a physician's MD* indicate that the physician is a fellow of a particular college and very probably a diplomate of the board in that specialty. A comprehensive listing of all diplomates of the various specialty boards is published in the *Directory of Medical Specialists*, available in some libararies (the 17th edition is the latest).

*Some doctors use the initials PC following the MD. The initials PC do not in any way signify professional qualification or achievement. They stand for professional corporation; the laws of many states permit physicians to incorporate their practices.

195

American Board certification usually means that the physician's practice is restricted to the specialty. And, from the doctor's point of view, American Board certification is becoming increasingly important. In order to get prestigious university or hospital affiliations, from which patient referrals are derived, specialists usually need to be board-certified. Board certification is also important to them because of the higher fees paid to specialists by insurance companies, workmen's compensation boards, and other "third party" bill-payers.

Patients should be aware that any licensed physician can legally practice any surgical or medical specialty. Initials such as those noted above can offer reassurance that a physician has adequate training in a specialty. Such identification can be quite helpful to the prospective patient, who should not assume that hospital affiliation is necessarily equated with professional ability.

During the first quarter of this century the slow rate of change in medical knowledge made it possible for a general practitioner to provide patients with care consistent with existing knowledge in most medical fields. Then began the scientific advances that have escalated in the last twenty years. Because no doctor can possibly keep up with the rate of advance in the entire field of medicine, the tendency is to gain expertise in small segments of the field. Even in the area of surgery, the multiplicity of new techniques constantly being introduced is forcing surgeons to restrict themselves to certain parts of the body.

For today's doctor, hospitals are both workshops and centers for continuing education in the specialty area. At the hospital a physician's medical knowledge is reinforced and expanded through conferences, discussions, and association with colleagues, as well as through experience with patients.

Continuing education is the hallmark of a good "teaching" hospital—a hospital that has established a formal program for training house staff (resident physicians in their first several years out of medical school). Particularly during daily hospital rounds, practicing doctors and house staff share opinions, knowledge of recent developments, and experience.

Because continuing education is so crucial to the professional advancement of many doctors, staff positions at a teaching hospital are sought after. And to maintain good teaching capabilities and reputation, hospitals usually insist that prospective staff members be well qualified.

Within the medical profession, such organizations as the American Academy of Family Physicians (AAFP) are trying to revitalize general practice. The AAFP requirements for membership make mandatory one of the following: three years of approved graduate training, two years of graduate training plus two years of general practice, or one year of graduate training plus three years of general practice during which the applicant must complete 150 hours of approved education. After being accepted for membership, all who wish to continue as active members are then required to complete 150 hours of accredited postgraduate study every three years. There are now more than 30,000 members, plus an additional 5,400 student affiliates. Osteopathic physicians (see below) are also eligible for membership.

In 1970, medicine appeared to have come full circle when the specialty of generalists called family practice received board certification status, and the American Board of Family Practice conducted its first certifying examination. By the end of 1975 there were 7,015 physicians certified in family practice. More than three-quarters of these physicians are also members of the AAFP.

In addition, many state and local medical societies have set up sections on general practice, and many medical schools have established professorships and departments of family practice. It appears likely that these efforts may offset to some extent the trend toward specialization.

Undoubtedly, family practice will occupy an increasingly important place in medicine in the United States. While the new specialty grows, many patients turn to the internist for the provision of primary medical care. An internist is a physician with postgraduate training in the broad field of internal medicine—that is, in all areas of medicine except surgical, obstetric, and pediatric practice. By the end of 1975, 30,372 diplomates were certified by the American Board of Internal Medicine. In addition, there are thousands of board-eligible internists.

Within internal medicine there are various subspecialty areas, each with its own subspecialty board. These areas include allergy, cardiology, endocrinology, gastroenterology, hematology, nephrology, oncology, pulmonary disease, and rheumatology.

Whether certified or eligible, the internists' training and expertise in internal medicine should make them particularly capable of dealing with heart and kidney disease, diabetes, and arthritis, as well as disorders affecting the blood and endocrine systems. Their training should also increase their interest in the occupational, emotional, and social aspects of disease. Because of this broad training and interest, internists are usually well qualified to serve as personal physicians and family medical advisers. They can take care of most common disorders themselves, but refer patients to other specialists when necessary.

The fact that doctors are board-certified or board-eligible internists or that they're certified in family practice or members of the AAFP does not automatically ensure care of the highest quality. But the odds *are* in the patient's favor.

In several states such chances are enhanced somewhat by specific requirements physicians must meet in order to remain in good standing in their profession. Although all doctors must be licensed by their respective state boards of medical examiners, in most states renewal of licenses is a mere formality. As of this writing, only New Mexico makes renewal of the license to practice medicine contingent upon a prescribed amount of postgraduate study. In fourteen other states—Alaska, Arizona, California, Colorado, Illinois, Kansas, Kentucky, Michigan, Minnesota, Nebraska, Ohio, Utah, Washington, and Wisconsin—the medical examiners have been authorized to require evidence of continuing medical education for reregistration but have never implemented the policy.

Most state and county medical societies have been slow to support mandatory postgraduate education in medicine. In fourteen states the medical societies have endorsed the principle of requiring continuing medical education as a condition of membership renewal. As of this writing, however, the medical societies of only four states—Arizona, New Jersey, Oregon (which pioneered the concept), and Pennsylvania—actually have such a procedure in operation. (Alabama, Florida, Kansas, Maine, Massachusetts, Minnesota, Montana, New York, North Carolina, and Vermont are the ten states whose medical societies have endorsed the principle.) California's medical society has a unique program with even more stringent standards than the typical mandatory requirement of 150 hours of graduate study over three years—but it is voluntary.

All twenty-two medical specialty boards have now gone on record as supporting periodic reexamination as a means of encouraging high levels of professionalism. As of this writing, only one—the American Board of Family Practice —has actually required mandatory examinations at regular intervals for continued certification. The first certifying examination for family practice was held in 1970. In 1976 those who qualified in 1970 could once again qualify for certification by taking a second examination. None of the other specialty boards has yet followed suit, although the American Board of Internal Medicine prepared a *voluntary* examination offered to internists by the American College of Physicians in 1974.

CU endorses the efforts of various medical societies and of state boards of medical examiners to require postgraduate study for practicing physicians. Until better mechanisms are devised to enhance the quality of the medical professional, CU believes that the most effective way to cull the incompetent is periodic, mandatory examination.

Another category of health professional available for personal medical care is the osteopathic physician. The American Osteopathic Association claims that "diagnostic and therapeutic methods applied to [the musculoskeletal] system make osteopathic medicine today's most comprehensive and complete approach to man's health problems." CU's medical consultants, who are MDs, do not agree with that statement. Apart from such claims, however, osteopathy is becoming increasingly recognized by organized medicine, both on national and state levels. Graduates of schools of osteopathy (there are ten in the United States) receive an education similar in many respects to that offered by medical schools.

There are currently about 15,500 osteopathic physicians, approximately 75 percent of whom are in family practice. As with MDs, doctors of osteopathy (DOs) may become certified in the various specialties by taking qualifying examinations (administered by one of the American Osteopathic Boards). Most of the twenty-two medical specialty boards also now permit osteopaths to qualify for certification examinations; prominent exceptions are the American Board of Surgery and several boards related to surgery.

Osteopaths are *not* to be confused with chiropractors, who are, in the opinion of CU's medical consultants, no substitute for medical professionals. (See our report on chiropractic, page 228.)

Even if you would like to confine your search for a personal doctor to an internist, you may not be able to locate one who can take on new patients. In that case, you may find the personal medical adviser you are seeking in a general practitioner—one with a limited practice who, like an internist, does not deliver babies or perform major surgery.

The category of ideal personal doctor, therefore, in addition to the internist, includes the general practitioner who neither performs major surgery nor practices obstetrics and who is on the staff of an accredited hospital, preferably one that is also a teaching hospital.

How do you set out to find a personal physician? Ideally, the pertinent professional facts about *all* physicians in a community should be readily available to every consumer. Unfortunately, they rarely are. A Washington-based public-interest organization, the Health Research Group, attempted to provide the facts by publishing *A Consumer's Directory of Prince George's County (Md.) Doctors.* Many of the doctors refused to respond to a questionnaire and the Health Research Group met with little practical success. But it gained a fund of experience that organized consumers elsewhere can put to good use. For a questionnaire that may help nonprofit groups to develop local directories of physicians, see pages 685-691 of the September 1974 CONSUMER REPORTS (available at your public library or for $1 from Back Issue Dept., Consumers Union, Orangeburg, N.Y. 10962). Meanwhile, until consumer groups can supply you with objective data about doctors in your community, we offer these proposals for finding a personal physician now.

Recommendations

If you are moving to a new location, the simplest way to choose a doctor is to ask a physician whose judgment you trust to recommend one. The physician may be acquainted with doctors in your new area or may be able to verify for you the qualifications of possible family doctors. Otherwise, after you have moved, check with the nearest accredited hospital. Ask the hospital for a list of internists or general practitioners who are on its staff as attending physicians. If a medical school is situated near your new home town, a telephone inquiry may produce the names of internists or qualified family doctors on the faculty who practice in your community. A friend or relative whose judgment you respect and who knows your likes and dislikes may often prove to be a valuable lead to a new family doctor. The county medical society will provide names of internists and general practitioners in your immediate vicinity—more official, but not much more informative, than what you find in the Yellow Pages.

With a list of qualified candidates, you can make a telephone survey to find one who seems suitable. It would make sense to start with those whose offices are close to where you live, for convenience as well as prompt care in an emergency. Let the doctor know that you are selecting a personal physician and do not hesitate to ask questions about fees, hospital affiliations, attitude toward home calls, and any other matters that concern you. Having chosen the key physician, you can then expect help in selecting specialists.

Check also to see if there's a nearby prepaid comprehensive medical service plan that could provide the services of a qualified internist or family doctor. Known as HMOs (health maintenance organizations), these plans offer subscribers a variety of medical services for a fixed monthly fee paid in advance. (See page 207 for our report on HMOs.) Some consumers may find the HMO style of health-care delivery more to their taste than traditional fee-for-service care, and possibly more economical.

No matter what process you have used, the physician you select could later turn out to be unacceptable. Personalities may clash, or you may object to a lack of candor or the fees charged. The doctor may refuse to call in consultants or may be too impatient to discuss details of your case with you. The office may be so poorly organized that messages do not get through. Under such circumstances, it might be wise to look around for another doctor.

On the other hand, someone who changes doctors for trivial reasons rarely benefits from an endless search for the ideal doctor. The chronic doctor shopper may be a greater loser than the patient who can overlook one or two uncomfortable encounters with the office bureaucracy or an isolated brusque moment with the doctor.

How to Judge a Hospital

When you choose a personal physician, you choose more than a lone practitioner. You also choose the hospital or hospitals that the doctor uses for patient care. But hospitals differ sharply in quality of care and in scope of services. In judging physicians, consider very carefully the hospitals to which they admit patients. And in judging a hospital, ask these three main questions:

1. Is the hospital accredited? Roughly two-thirds of the 7,200 general hospitals in the United States are accredited by the Joint Commission on Accreditation of Hospitals (JCAH). Accreditation does not guarantee that a hospital is first-rate, but it does reduce the likelihood of substandard medical care and a hazardous physical plant.

If a hospital wants to be accredited, it must conform to basic standards in its operation and in the delivery of care and services. Its conformity is evaluated by means of a detailed questionnaire and an on-site inspection by a JCAH survey team. Interested consumers can participate in the evaluation by requesting a hearing before the on-site survey team.

A hospital given JCAH accreditation usually displays its certificate in the lobby. But if you are uncertain whether a hospital is accredited, you can find out by asking the hospital's administrators or by writing to the Office of Public Information of the JCAH, 875 North Michigan Avenue, Chicago, Ill. 60611.

2. Is it a "teaching" hospital? As noted earlier in the report, a "teaching" hospital has a formal program for training medical personnel. The higher the level of training, the higher the level of medical services a hospital is likely to provide.

The best indicator of a good teaching program is affiliation with a medical school. (You can find out if a hospital is so affiliated by writing to the Office of Public Affairs, American Hospital Association, 840 North Lake Shore Drive, Chicago, Ill. 60611.) Such hospitals are likely to have available the services of qualified family doctors and a full range of specialists. They often have full-time staff physicians in charge of key departments. And they attract many good young physicians who want residency training in specialties.

But medical schools and their affiliated hospitals are not spread evenly across the United States. You might not have easy access to any of them. You may obtain somewhat similar benefits, however, from a nonaffiliated hospital approved for residency training in medicine and surgery. The next best choice is a hospital that has a nursing school or training programs for ancillary personnel, such as laboratory or X-ray technicians.

3. **Who "owns" the hospital?** Is it a voluntary, nonprofit community hospital? Or is it a privately owned, proprietary hospital? Or is it a third type, a public institution sponsored by the municipal, county, state, or federal government? Hospitals within each category vary widely in quality. But in the judgment of CU's medical consultants, the voluntary hospital is usually the patient's best choice. In selecting a doctor, consider affiliation with a voluntary hospital as a plus factor.

Voluntary hospitals are nonprofit community institutions functioning under religious or other voluntary auspices. They generally offer good medical facilities and competent staff. In the best of them, there are strict provisions for inspection, evaluation, and control of the medical activities of affiliated doctors.

Proprietary hospitals are commercial establishments. They are, of course, intended to help sick people, but they are also intended to make a profit. The physical surroundings are often plush, and the food may be tastier than that in voluntary hospitals. But, on the whole, proprietary institutions exert less control over the medical qualifications and activities of their affiliated physicians.

Most proprietary hospitals concentrate on illnesses that can be treated relatively simply. For procedures such as traction, hernia operations, and routine obstetrical deliveries, a JCAH-accredited proprietary hospital may be entirely adequate. But the lack of certain sophisticated equipment and services may make some of those hospitals poor places to be for complicated illnesses.

Government-supported hospitals, some very large and some quite small, share a distinctive mission—they will provide medical care for the indigent (though any sick person, regardless of need, may be admitted to such hospitals). In general, they offer good medical services. In those that are affiliated with medical schools, the facilities and staff may be superb. But government-sponsored institutions may fall behind voluntary hospitals in such matters as comfortable accommodations. And they may sometimes be compelled to curtail services when government budgets are cut.

Are Health Maintenance Organizations the Answer to Your Medical Needs?

Organizations that offer a broad range of medical services for an annual fee have been around since 1929 in the United States. But until recent years, relatively few people had access to them. You had to live in a particular location or work for a specific employer to join one.

Today that situation is changing. Stoked by federal funds and the government's official blessing, health maintenance organizations—HMOs for short—are emerging as an alternative to traditional, fee-for-service medicine for a growing number of Americans.

What is an HMO? And more important, how does it compare with the familiar form of medical service most of us grew up with?

A typical HMO assembles under one roof a number of health services for its enrolled members. Instead of charging a fee for each service, the HMO collects a lump sum in advance from subscribers (or their employers). That sum is supposed to pay for comprehensive health care by the

HMO's physicians. HMO, then, is another name for prepaid group practice or group health.

The best known HMO is the Kaiser Foundation Health Plan (usually referred to as Kaiser-Permanente). Its roots go back to 1933, when a small group of doctors was retained to care for workers on a construction project in the Mojave Desert. The plan was gradually expanded to cover Kaiser employes in other locations, then opened to the public after World War II. The Kaiser Foundation Health Plan now serves some 2.7 million patients in California, Colorado, Hawaii, Ohio, Oregon, and Washington.

Group health plans sprang up elsewhere in the 1930s and 1940s, usually in response to the needs of an organized group of patients. But by 1970 there were still only twenty-five such plans in the entire country. Development had been slow in part because the canons of medical ethics prevented plans from advertising, which hindered recruitment and limited public awareness of the plans. More important, though, was the opposition of organized medicine.

Medical associations had promoted passage of state laws that discouraged prepaid medicine. The laws prohibited the practice of medicine by corporations and required prepaid plans to invite a majority of physicians in a locality to participate (an impossible requirement). And they required the plans to maintain large sums of money as reserves.

County medical societies refused membership to group-health physicians and prevented them from gaining admission privileges at hospitals, from qualifying for specialty board examinations, and even from attending postgraduate courses. These roadblocks were removed only after the United States Department of Justice intervened. The Supreme Court in 1943 upheld a suit filed by the Justice Department, ruling that the actions of the American Medical

Association and the Washington, D.C., Medical Society against a Washington-based plan were an unlawful restraint of trade.

The court decision and subsequent actions by some state courts improved the atmosphere for prepaid medicine during the 1950s and 1960s. But the HMO idea didn't catch fire until the 1970s, when government officials seized on it as a possible solution to rapidly rising health costs.

Backed by some government money and encouragement, the number of HMOs increased sevenfold between 1970 and 1974. There are now 175 prepaid health-care plans with just over six million people enrolled in thirty-five states and the District of Columbia. And as a result of a federal law enacted in December 1973—and amended in October 1976—many more people will have the opportunity to choose between a prepaid plan and traditional fee-for-service practice.

The 1973 law authorized the Department of Health, Education, and Welfare (HEW) to disburse $325 million to aid formation of new HMOs and to assist existing programs through grants, contracts, and loans. The act also superseded restrictive state laws that had impeded HMOs from forming and flourishing. A third aspect of the 1973 law, implemented in October 1975, was aimed at increasing consumer access to HMOs through mandating so-called dual option: a requirement that certain employers of twenty-five or more people offer as part of employe health benefits the option of membership in a federally qualified HMO, should there be one available in the area. As of December 1976, however, only twenty-two HMOs were deemed qualified by HEW under the provisions of the 1973 act—with three more HMOs in the final stages of qualification.

To become qualified under the 1973 act, an HMO had to agree to base its premiums on a "community" rating rather than on an "experience" rating. A community rate includes the more costly medical needs of the poor and the elderly and is relatively high. An experience rate is usually based on the medical needs of an employe group (relatively healthy, by definition) and is usually lower.

An HMO also had to agree to conduct yearly enrollments that allowed anyone in the community to join without facing restrictions on the amount of care provided for preexisting illness. Furthermore, to be qualified, an HMO would have to offer coverage that included not only typical HMO benefits but also short-term mental health services, treatment and referral services for alcoholism and drug abuse, therapeutic X-ray, home health care, family planning and infertility services, preventive dental care for children, children's eye examinations, medical social services, and health education programs for subscribers.

The combination of community rating, open enrollment, and a rich benefits package placed qualifying HMOs at a severe cost disadvantage under dual option. Insurance companies were not required to meet any of those conditions, which would have raised their premium rates. HEW estimated in 1974 that the HMO benefits package would cost a minimum of $70 a month for a family. When the 1973 law was enacted, $70 was the extreme upper limit of HMO charges—and almost twice what the typical employer contributed toward health insurance premiums. That meant that employes who chose the HMO option might have to pay sizable sums out of their own pockets to make up the difference. (The law did not require an employer to increase the company contribution.)

Under these circumstances, employes most likely to go for the HMO option would be those with the greatest medical needs. That's called adverse selection. And adverse selection combined with open enrollment would tend to flood an HMO with the sickest members of the community, thus threatening the solvency of the prepaid program.

Not surprisingly, relatively few HMOs sought to be accepted by HEW as qualified under the 1973 law. HMOs without federal certification, should they want to vie for employe business, would have to compete against lower-cost coverage for the *conventional* insurance slot in dual option. Without designation as qualified, prepaid health plans could not be eligible for the HMO slot. That, in turn, meant that many workers, despite the 1973 law, would continue to have only one choice of coverage for some years to come—conventional health insurance.

To improve the outlook for HMOs, Congress acted in 1976 to amend the 1973 law and put prepaid plans on a more competitive footing with insurance companies. The lawmakers scaled back the requirements leading to qualified status in several significant ways.

For example, preventive health services, which an HMO must offer to its members, were redefined to include only immunization, well-child care from birth, children's eye and ear examinations, periodic health examinations for adults, voluntary family planning services, and infertility services. Crucial language in the 1976 amendments concerning supplemental health services substituted the permissive words, "the organization may provide," for the previous compulsory "shall provide." This put in the optional category such potentially costly items as vision, dental, and mental health services beyond basic preventive care, and facilities for intermediate and long-term care as well as rehabilitation services.

The financial impact of open enrollment was lessened by limiting the requirement to an HMO in operation for five years or with an enrollment of fifty thousand or without a deficit in its most recent fiscal year. (Even then, the requirement could be sidestepped if it jeopardized an HMO's financial health.) What's more, open enrollment now would generally mean that an HMO need not enroll more than 3 percent of its net increase in enrollment during the prior fiscal year.

Also a target of the 1976 amendments was the controversial commmunity rating requirement. Among other changes, newly qualified HMOs that had been in operation prior to HEW designation as qualified would be allowed forty-eight months to meet the requirement that their contracts be community rated. Dual option was also facilitated by a clause providing that only twenty-five employes need live in the service area of a qualified HMO to make mandatory the offer of an HMO option.

Many politicians favor HMO development because it offers a potential solution to several problems of traditional medicine and health insurance—problems they are being pressed to solve. One problem is the difficulty many people have in finding satisfactory medical services. Another is the fragmentation of those services: widely separated office locations, lack of easy communication among specialists treating the same patient, and the scattering of a patient's medical and hospital records in several locations.

A third problem is the high cost of medical services. Typical health insurance policies limit coverage of outpatient and preventive services but richly reimburse hospitalization. That encourages use of high-cost hospital facilities when a doctor's office might serve as well—and also cost less. What's more, the fee-for-service structure creates incentives for some doctors to provide unnecessary or questionable services, particularly when an insurance company will pay for some or all of the bill, no questions asked, and simply pass on the cost in the form of higher premiums. Under such circumstances, the more services doctors provide, the more they earn—whether the patient really needs all the services or not.

In theory, an HMO addresses those three problems. By joining an HMO, the subscriber gains access to a team of doctors. Besides primary-care physicians (internists, general practitioners, pediatricians), there are, depending on the HMO's size, various additional specialists available, such as radiologists, surgeons, obstetricians-gynecologists, neurologists, and the like. The HMO guarantees around-the-clock medical care 365 days a year. A primary-care physician coordinates all of the patient's health care, including referral to specialists outside the organization if necessary. (The HMO, not the subscriber, pays the outside specialist's bill.)

The fragmentation of traditional medicine is replaced by one-stop health care. The HMO's team of doctors, nurses, laboratory technicians, and administrative staff works together in a single building, which includes laboratory and diagnostic facilities. There are treatment rooms for minor surgical procedures that might otherwise require hospitalization. A patient's complete medical record is stored in a single location. When hospitalization is needed, the HMO arranges and pays for it. Many HMOs even have their own pharmacies.

In financial structure, an HMO also differs markedly from fee-for-service practice and traditional health insurance. The HMO sells what amounts to a guarantee that it will *provide*, not just pay for, a stated range of health services. The fee for a family is roughly between $840 and $1,080 a year ($70 to $90 per month), depending on the extent of services provided and the area of the country. Covered services typically include all medical and surgical care, diagnostic laboratory tests and X-rays, out-of-area benefits, and hospitalization. The fee for a family is the same amount regardless of the number of children.

HMO physicians are on salary, or its equivalent, which removes any incentive for them to run up unnecessary services. The HMO's economic incentive is to *prevent* illness—or at least detect and treat it early—because a single day in the hospital will cost the equivalent of a few months of the subscriber's fees. For the subscriber, in turn, medical outlays are predictable because most essential services are covered by the regular fee. And the HMO's broad physician and hospital benefits largely remove the financial threat of catastrophic illness.

An HMO puts particular emphasis on outpatient and preventive care. HMO proponents are convinced that traditional medicine wastes money by overemphasizing hospital use. By contrast, a health plan that stresses prevention and early detection of disease should, in theory, keep its members healthier—or at least hospitalized less. Money saved on hospitalization can then go to finance preventive care that conventional health insurance often does not cover. Or so the argument runs for HMOs.

Does the idea work in practice?

The University of California School of Public Health studied whether patients in two established HMOs in Southern California received more preventive services than did fee-for-service patients. Hospital and medical records were traced for physical checkups, well-child examinations, Pap smears, chest X-rays, routine rectal examinations, blood tests for syphilis, and immunizations. The investigators computed a "preventive service index," which ranged from zero (no service) to 1.0 (maximum provision of preventive services). The higher the number, the more services a patient received. The index was .384 for commercial insurance subscribers, .404 for Blue Cross-Blue Shield members, and .452 for HMO patients.

Another study reviewed the frequency of physical examinations among a controlled population in Alameda County, Calif. Fifty-eight percent of the men enrolled in a local Kaiser-Permanente plan had such a checkup during the preceding year, whereas only 43 to 46 percent of those with conventional policies had one. Among women, the scores were 63 percent for HMO members versus 49 to 57 percent for conventional insurance subscribers.

While HMO members may receive more preventive services than fee-for-service patients, does it help them stay healthier or live longer? Two studies involving the Health Insurance Plan of New York (HIP), a large health maintenance organization, have examined this question.

One compared HIP subscribers with private patients in terms of premature birth rates and perinatal mortality (infant deaths at birth or during the first month of life). The prematurity rate per 100 live births was 5.5 for white HIP subscribers, versus 6.0 for a matched group of private patients. Among nonwhites the spread was even greater: 8.8 in HIP, 10.8 for private patients. The perinatal mortality rate per 1,000 births and fetal deaths was 22.7 for white HIP patients, against 27.3 among white private patients. Nonwhite statistics were 33.7 for HIP, 43.8 for private patients. The differences, which were statistically significant, clearly favored HIP.

The second HIP study compared death rates at the other end of the life span. A group of Old Age Assistance recipients who obtained care from HIP were matched with a similar group who received care under the traditional fee-for-service welfare system. In the first year, mortality was virtually identical among both groups. During the next eighteen months, however, the yearly mortality rate was 7.8 per 100 persons in the HIP group and 8.8 for the others —a difference of 13 per cent, and a clear edge again for HIP.

Studies have consistently found less hospital use and fewer surgical procedures among HMO patients. The most definitive study involved 8 million federal employes and beneficiaries who had a choice between conventional health insurance or an available HMO. HEW compared the number of days per year each group of a thousand persons spent in the hospital under the two types of medical care.

Those with Blue Cross-Blue Shield coverage averaged 924 days; those with other insurance, 987 days. But HMO members spent only 422 days—a hospitalization rate less than half that of the others. Compared with HMO members, federal subscribers to the "Blue" plans underwent twice as much surgery of all types—including three times as many tonsillectomies and twice as many gynecological operations. Tonsillectomies and such gynecological operations as hysterectomies are precisely those procedures that, critics have charged, benefit some fee-for-service doctors more often than they benefit their patients.

The money HMOs save on hospital costs can result in lower overall medical expenses for subscribers. A California study showed that total medical costs for one year among families subscribing to two HMOs in the Los Angeles area were $124 less than those for families with Blue Cross-Blue Shield. In 1974, members of an HMO at Columbia, Md., purchased a representative package of medical and hospital coverage for $169 less than it would have cost with a typical insurance policy.

HMOs offer other possible advantages that proponents hope to substantiate. It is argued, for example, that HMO members—because they have already paid in advance—are more likely to seek medical attention for illness in its early stages, thus avoiding needless hospitalization stemming from neglect. Proponents also claim that the HMO's centralized structure should save money through economies of scale—in bulk purchase of drugs and other supplies, for example.

Emphasis on a coordinated approach to health care may also make HMOs ideal places to provide health education in nutrition, cancer detection, and similar subjects. The Group Health Cooperative of Puget Sound and the Georgetown University Community Health Plan of Washington, D.C., have run impressive subscriber-education programs. The 1973 HMO law required HMOs seeking federal qualification to offer health education programs for their subscribers.

HMOs, of course, are not without drawbacks, theoretical and real. If the financial incentive in traditional medicine is to provide too many services, the financial incentive for an HMO could be to provide too few—to scrimp on care and pocket the difference. Fortunately, there are checks against such scrimping.

First of all, subscribers would leave the plan (which is precisely what's happened in California's "Medicaid mills," discussed below). A second check is the malpractice suits that scrimping invites. A third is that the neglect of basic care could cause hospitalization to soar, which would drain those theoretical profits. In actuality, with the exception of California's Medicaid experience, studies of HMO performance do not show scrimping to be a problem.

Another drawback of the HMO concept is that it limits members' choice of physician and sometimes their choice of hospital. Covered care is from the HMO's panel of physicians only, except when a nonaffiliated specialist must be called in. Joining an HMO means giving up one's fee-for-service doctors, unless you pay them out of pocket. And joining some HMOs, such as Kaiser-Permanente, or Compcare of Milwaukee, means using only that group's hospital.

Those limitations are sometimes more theoretical than

real, however. In many parts of the United States, particularly in rural communities, one's choice of physician or hospital is limited anyway. And freedom of choice doesn't mean much when the demand for doctors exceeds the supply.

A third disadvantage can be limitations that an HMO places on reimbursement for illness or accident outside its service area. Although HMOs customarily provide a measure of out-of-area coverage, some prefer to treat patients as quickly as possible in their own hospitals. The reason is financial. An HMO controls its own costs; but it can't control costs in a hospital or clinic many miles away where a subscriber is receiving treatment that the HMO pays for. Having to interrupt travel to return to one's home HMO for treatment could prove inconvenient.

A fourth possible disadvantage can be impersonal care: long waits for nonemergency appointments and an atmosphere resembling, to some people, that of public clinics. Large HMOs are indeed complex bureaucracies, and their needs don't always match those of their clients. A measure of impersonality is perhaps inevitable because HMOs insist on efficient use of their physicians' time and on rational procedures geared to save money (scheduling doctor appointments like airline reservations, as one former Kaiser official put it).

The most common complaint of HMO subscribers concerns the doctor-patient relationship. The primary-care physician isn't always available or may seem too busy or not personally interested, or may delegate work to nurses or paramedical workers when the patient might prefer the doctor's personal ministrations.

About one-third of the members of two HMOs surveyed did not consider their plan physician as their "family" or "regular" doctor and purchased additional medical services outside the plan. Four out of ten subscribers to Community Health of Detroit, for instance, used outside doctors over a three-year period. Yet, of those who did, 68 percent reported continued satisfaction with the plan.

But HMOs haven't cornered the market on impersonality. Similar problems exist, of course, in fee-for-service medicine. Doctors can be booked up months in advance for physical checkups, and the atmosphere of a large fee-for-service practice can be impersonal too. In any office in which a number of physicians share space, equipment, and staff, the traditional one-to-one relationship between doctor and patient can also become submerged in bureaucracy.

Overall, a number of surveys indicate that the majority of HMO subscribers are satisfied with their plans. The studies consistently turn up about 10 percent who are clearly dissatisfied. But that experience still compares favorably with traditional practice. According to the University of California School of Public Health, approximately 20 percent of fee-for-service patients are clearly dissatisfied with the care they receive.

Variations on the HMO Theme

Organized medicine's answer to the HMO is the medical foundation, called an individual practice association (IPA), the best known of which are two in California—San Joaquin and Sacramento—and one in suburban Portland, Ore. (the Physicians Association of Clackamas County).

An IPA is often an offshoot of a county medical society. It collects an annual fee that covers a subscriber's hospitalization and basic medical services. The fee is comparable to that of a typical HMO.

Unlike the typical HMO, however, an IPA does not contract to provide services at a one-stop health facility. Subscribers must arrange their own medical care from doctors belonging to the IPA. The doctors, in turn, bill the IPA on a fee-for-service basis. If the IPA runs short of money, participating doctors don't collect their full fee, and they can't bill subscribers for the difference.

An IPA, in short, is the financing half of an HMO, a sort of super Blue Cross-Blue Shield. It does not offer coordinated services at one location, but it does guarantee subscribers more predictable costs. While it may go under the *name* of HMO, it does not engage in group practice the way a typical HMO does. The dual option of the 1973 HMO law (see page 209) may also apply to an IPA that is available in an area and qualified according to HEW standards.

Blue Cross and Blue Shield, according to HEW, are expanding efforts to offer their members an HMO option and are currently involved in sponsoring more than a hundred HMOs. One early program in eleven Wisconsin counties permits patients to sign up with a participating primary-care physician, who assumes responsibility for providing and coordinating all medical care in exchange for a fixed annual fee paid by the program. The primary-care physician must approve all referrals to specialists and all hospital admissions; specialist and hospital fees are billed separately.

Another variety of HMO bears mention, primarily for its difference in quality. Heavy criticism has been leveled at the prepaid health plans that began to spring up in 1971 to serve Medicaid recipients in California. Former governor Ronald Reagan had predicted that the plans would save the state millions of dollars by slashing what he claimed was the overuse of traditional medical services by welfare recipients. Instead, the plans appear to be highly successful in wasting the taxpayers' money, as well as in scrimping on services.

By 1974, there were fifty-two prepaid plans in California

enrolling some 240,000 Medicaid recipients. That year the California Auditor General reported the results of an examination of the fifteen largest plans. Of the $56.5 million the state paid to the fifteen plans in 1971 through 1973, only 48 percent went for medical services. An extraordinarily high 52 percent went for various administrative expenses (data processing, enrollment, rent and overhead, and the salaries and expenses of plan officials).

Such administrative costs should never exceed 15 percent of income, even in the costly startup phase of an HMO, according to an official of the Group Health Association of America (GHAA). Typically, they're between 5 and 10 percent for GHAA-member HMOs.

HEW investigated the California Medicaid mills in 1974 and reported "abuses in the marketing of prepaid health care services, failure in the delivery of promised services, and deficiencies in state monitoring practices." Citizens have picketed several of the plans in protest over high-pressure recruitment tactics and broken promises. Congressional committees have held hearings too, most recently in November 1976. Federal and California health officials agree that the worst abuses will be controlled once new regulations become effective in 1977 requiring each HMO under contract to the state to meet federal standards for qualification.

Evaluating an HMO

HMOs vary in a number of ways—some important, some not. There are large urban programs with hundreds of thousands of subscribers and small rural ones with just a thousand or so members. A few own their own hospitals; many do not. Some operate from a single clinic; others have several locations in a community. Some have pharmacies at each of their locations; some have no pharmacy at all.

Some are profit-making enterprises; many others are non-profit corporations. The most important differences among HMOs are reviewed below as a guide to possible selection. **Staff qualifications.** A well-trained, qualified staff of physicians is naturally a prime requisite. It's preferable if an HMO's physicians are *board-certified* in their specialty areas or are at least *board-eligible* (see page 195). A 1974 survey conducted by the GHAA for the federal government found that only nineteen of forty-five HMOs sampled required board-certification or board-eligibility of their doctors.

Another favorable sign is a staff that has teaching responsibilities on a hospital faculty, which often indicates a continuing interest in medical education and developments. Doctors at eleven of the forty-five HMOs surveyed by the GHAA engaged in such teaching. Absence of teaching responsibility should not automatically count against an HMO, however. Rural health maintenance organizations that are distant from medical teaching centers can't be expected to meet that criterion. (For a full discussion of how to evaluate a doctor's credentials, see "How to Find a Doctor for Yourself," page 194.)

Quality assurance programs. Every HMO should have a formal program in which doctors regularly review one another's work. The 1974 GHAA survey found that thirty-two of the forty-five HMOs in its survey had such programs. At that time, a quality assessment committee at the Group Health Association of Washington, D.C., for example, reviewed the records of forty patients every two weeks to check doctor performance. Kaiser-Permanente sent a team of physicians from one of its medical centers to another each month to review records; findings were reported to the entire staff. A special committee at the East Baltimore Medical Plan reviewed medical records weekly for continuity of care, omissions, and errors in diagnosis or patient management.

Doctor-patient ratios. Group-health specialists recommend that an HMO have at least one primary-care doctor for every thousand to twelve hundred subscribers. Fewer physicians than that could mean long waits and compromised care. Health officials whom CU consulted say that minimum staffing requirements are usually met and often exceeded. Even so, CU suggests you check on the doctor-patient ratio.

Consumer participation. Subscribers should have an effective voice in such policy matters as the kinds of services provided, child-care arrangements, and the location and hours of clinics. GHAA statistics are encouraging. Thirty-seven of the forty-five HMOs surveyed had either subscriber representatives on the board of directors, a consumer advisory council, or a formal grievance committee that included consumer representatives.

The least satisfactory grievance procedure was that of the Western Clinic in Tacoma, Wash. The business manager settled complaints with no provision for appeal. The most satisfactory procedure was that typified by the HMO at St. Louis Park Medical Center in Minnesota, which had a formal mechanism for appealing to the consumer advisory board, and then to the board of directors. If necessary, the appeal could even go to arbitration for resolution.

The Group Health Cooperative of Puget Sound offers prospective subscribers the names of members who are willing to discuss the plan's service. Any plan that won't provide such references, with appropriate safeguards for members' privacy, should be considered suspect.

Other considerations. Even if an HMO scores high in all of the foregoing categories, it may still be no bargain if it's hard to get to. An HMO with only a single location can be inconvenient if you live across town; one with branches can be a boon. For some patients, convenient access to public transportation or parking may be important.

Most HMOs are nonprofit corporations. Some group health advocates argue that consumers should reject any HMO run for profit. They contend that it's immoral to profit from illness and that such plans might sacrifice the medical needs of subscribers for financial gain.

We don't think it's quite that simple. The medical profession by definition derives its livelihood from illness. Furthermore, some nonprofit HMOs have given entrepreneurs ample salaries and loans. (A $120,000 yearly salary was paid to the former director of one of those nominally "nonprofit" Medicaid mills in California.) Half of all nonprofit HMOs, in fact, have their own profit-making subsidiaries or subcontractors. And the economic consequences of substandard performance—subscriber resignation and malpractice suits—apply to profit and nonprofit HMOs alike.

While nonprofit HMOs with strong consumer participation are the most attractive choice in CU's view, the evidence is not yet persuasive for rejecting profit-making HMOs out of hand. If such a plan's qualifications are otherwise acceptable, it may merit your consideration.

Finally, one of the most important points to evaluate in an HMO is the benefits program it offers. Does that coverage include what you need?

HMOs uniformly cover diagnostic and X-ray services, hospitalization, and the services of physicians and surgeons. The fine-print exclusions of traditional health-insurance policies apply to HMOs as well. Usually excluded are cosmetic surgery, care in government-related institutions, organ transplants (except kidney), and usually convalescent, custodial, and rest care. Furthermore, most HMOs neither provide nor pay for speech and occupational therapy, orthopedic and prosthetic devices, hearing aids, eyeglasses, contact lenses, and blood or blood substitutes. And HMOs vary widely in their coverage of out-of-area hospitalization, prescription drugs, psychiatric care, maternity care, house calls, dental care, extended care in nursing homes, and copayments for service. Such coverage—or lack of it—could have a significant impact on your budget and should be examined carefully.

Out-of-area hospitalization. As noted earlier, HMOs are local organizations and may lack the coverage of national insurance plans. Depending on the HMO, coverage may range from full or partial payment to nothing at all.

Prescription drugs. Benefits range from all to nothing. Some HMOs provide prescription drugs at no charge to subscribers; others in the same area may offer no prescription coverage. In between are those that charge subscribers a flat fee per prescription or a percentage of the cost.

Psychiatric care. Here again, variation is wide. Some cover the equivalent of several months' psychiatric hospitalization and outpatient care as required. Other HMOs may limit psychiatric benefits to preliminary consultation and diagnosis.

Maternity care. This can be an important benefit for younger families. Most HMOs in the GHAA survey provided full maternity coverage after a reasonable waiting period. The Arizona Health Plan, on the other hand, charged a $500 deductible for a delivery. There was a similar copayment of $100 at the Columbia, Md., plan and $350 at CommuniCare of Los Angeles.

House calls. Like many of their counterparts in fee-for-service practice, physicians at some HMOs do not make house calls. A number of HMOs, however, provide house calls at no charge. Others charge; the fee can vary widely.

Dental care. Few plans at present provide this benefit.

Extended care. This benefit can be particularly important for middle-aged and elderly subscribers, who may require rehabilitative treatment for stroke or care in a skilled nursing home. Many HMOs, however, do not provide such coverage. Some, however, do provide up to a year or more of extended care benefits.

Copayments. Eleven of the forty-five HMOs in the GHAA survey charged subscribers small copayments for some of their basic services. Copayments serve two purposes. They lower subscription fees and may discourage frivolous use of HMO services. At the time of the GHAA survey, copayments of $2 per office visit were charged by ABC-HMO of Phoenix, Lovelace-Bataan of Albuquerque, and the Columbia, Md., plan. The fee was $1 at the Harvard and Kaiser plans. HMOs without copayments included those at Georgetown, Seattle, Yale, and the Labor Health Institute of St. Louis.

Recommendations

If the HMO idea sounds good to you, the easiest way to join one is through an employer or union group contract. That way there's likely to be no waiver or restriction of benefits for preexisting illness. Your employer may also pay part or all of the premium. The main drawback: Your choice will probably be limited to the HMO designated by your employer.

Individual memberships are also possible. If you can't locate an HMO, CU suggests two sources of information. The Group Health Association of America (1717 Massachusetts Avenue, N.W., Washington, D.C. 20036) will supply names of any member HMOs near you. The association's standards for membership offer a source of consumer protection. The other information source is the government's HMO program. Inquiries may be addressed to William J. McLeod, Office of Qualification and Compliance, HMO, Room 14A-35, Parklawn Building, 5600 Fishers Lane, Rockville, Md., 20857. That office has a record of all health maintenance organizations in your area that have received federal qualification.

Chiropractors: Healers or Quacks?

THE EIGHTY-YEAR WAR WITH SCIENCE

In a voice charged with emotion, Dr. Joseph Janse, president of the National College of Chiropractic, was addressing the hushed audience in the conference room.

"For me to stand here and exclaim or explain that I and my people, or those who preceded me, have never indulged in mishap or overclaim . . . would be dishonest.

". . . I am not, and we are not, necessarily proud of those that we are responsible for, and have to live with. But I do hope . . . this workshop will not deny the people of my profession the privilege of progress and ethics."

As on many previous occasions, Dr. Janse was responding to a challenge to chiropractic. But this occasion in February 1975 was different from the rest.

The conference, a "Workshop on the Research Status of Spinal Manipulative Therapy," was taking place in Bethesda, Md., at the National Institutes of Health (NIH). Never before had chiropractors participated in an international scientific conference in the United States, much less at the NIH, one of the world's foremost medical and biological research organizations. Throughout its eighty-year history, in fact, chiropractic has largely rejected or ignored advances in medical science fostered by agencies like the NIH. In turn, medical and government officials have generally branded chiropractic as "an unscientific cult" or "a significant hazard to the public." This time, however, the planning commission for the meeting—which was held in response to a Congressional mandate—included three chiropractors among its eight members.

The arrival of chiropractic in such a prestigious stronghold of science marked the latest in a series of developments that would seem to lend support to the chiropractor's demand for general recognition as a legitimate practitioner of the healing arts.

Despite opposition from organized medicine and the United States Public Health Service, chiropractors in 1973 won the right to render some services under both Medicare and Medicaid. Soon after, they achieved licensure in Louisiana and Mississippi, the last two holdouts among the fifty states. (The same period saw similar chiropractic gains in Canada.)

The crowning triumph for American chiropractors came in August 1974, when the United States Commissioner of Education recognized an accrediting agency for chiropractic colleges. This meant that colleges accredited by the Council on Chiropractic Education would have official national standing. Previously, degrees conferred by such institutions—for example, the Doctor of Chiropractic degree (DC)—were listed as "spurious" by the United States Office of Education. Recognition also meant that accredited chiropractic schools would be eligible for financial assistance under a variety of federal funding programs.

Chiropractic, in short, has made undeniable progress in

professional status and access to government-funded programs. Whether those gains mean equivalent progress for health care, however, is another question. In CU's view, the answer depends on whether chiropractic is a valid method of treatment or, as its critics contend, a form of quackery.

To explore that question, CU studied the current claims and practices of the profession to determine what chiropractic is and what potential benefits or harm a patient might experience. The resulting report is based on a six-month investigation that included an extensive review of chiropractic and medical literature, as well as the findings of pertinent national, state, and provincial government studies conducted in the United States and Canada over the last decade. CU visited three chiropractic colleges—Palmer, National, and Canadian Memorial—and also interviewed officials of the principal chiropractic associations, whose memberships include virtually all of the fifteen hundred chiropractors in active practice in the United States and some fourteen hundred chiropractors in Canada. CU also conducted interviews with American Medical Association representatives and with medical practitioners in orthopedics, physical medicine, neurosurgery, radiology, and other specialties. In the interest of objectivity, the assistance of CU's medical consultants was sought only for clarifying medical terminology or practices.

Chiropractic, which literally means "done by hand," originates from the theories of Daniel David Palmer, a tradesman who operated a "magnetic healing" studio in Davenport, Iowa, late in the nineteenth century. According to Palmer's writings, one of the passions of his life had been to discover the ultimate cause of disease—why one person should be ill while another person, "eating at the same table, working in the same shop," was spared illness. "This question," according to Palmer, "had worried thousands for centuries and was answered in September 1895."

The answer occurred to him, wrote Palmer, after treating a janitor he claimed was deaf. Palmer alleged that he restored the man's hearing by adjusting one of his vertebrae, the bony segments of the spine.

Apparently unaware that the nerves of hearing are entirely in the skull, Palmer theorized that he had relieved pressure on a spinal nerve that affected hearing. Adjusting the vertebrae, he decided, had removed interference with the nerve supply and thereby allowed the body's "Innate Intelligence" to effect a cure. Innate Intelligence, according to Palmer, was the "Soul, Spirit or Spark of Life," which he believed expressed itself through the nervous system to control the healing process. By supposedly impeding that expression, misaligned vertebrae were judged by Palmer as the cause of most disease.

In 1895, Palmer's emphasis on the spine raised fewer eyebrows among medical practitioners than it does today. Louis Pasteur had only recently demonstrated the plausibility of the germ theory of disease. And little more than a generation separated Palmer from many eminent physicians who had viewed the spine as the seat of innumerable human ills. It had been a common practice, in fact, to apply leeches, irritants, or even hot irons to tender sites along the spine as a treatment for various disorders.

By the end of the nineteenth century, however, such practices had waned. The scientific revolution that would shatter the boundaries of medicine in the twentieth century had already begun.

Osteopathy, which emerged a few years before chiropractic, adapted to the change. While retaining a separate identity—in part because of its use of manipulative therapy and its emphasis on the muscles and skeletal system—osteopathy gradually adopted the concepts and practices of orthodox medical science as well. Osteopathic students now receive training similar to that of medical students and earn a Doctor of Osteopathy (DO) degree (see page 200). In contrast, chiropractic maintained its allegiance to the nineteenth-century focus on the spine.

Some chiropractors still cling strictly to Palmer's theory that misalignments of the vertebrae—or "subluxations"—are the principal cause of disease. Such practitioners tend to advertise that chiropractic is crucial to good health. One recent ad, for instance, called vertebral subluxation "a killer of millions of people yearly." In the main, however, chiropractic recognizes other factors in illness. It does tend to assign bacteria and viruses a back seat, but it no longer ignores their existence. Essentially, it has modified Palmer's theories to accommodate some basic scientific realities. For example, modern chiropractic agrees with medicine that germs are factors in disease and that the body has inherent defense mechanisms against them. However, chiropractic stresses that *mechanical* disturbances of the nervous system are what impair the body's defenses. According to this theory, minor "off-centerings" of the vertebrae or pelvis might disturb nerve function and lower the body's resistance to germs. Structural misalignments, say chiropractors, may also disturb nerve impulses to the visceral organs, allegedly causing or aggravating such illnesses as heart disease, stomach ulcers, and diabetes.

"While many factors impair man's health, disturbances of the nervous system are among the most important," asserts the American Chiropractic Association (ACA). According to the association, almost anything can cause a mechanical subluxation that might trigger nerve disturbances: gravitational strain, asymmetrical activities and efforts, developmental defects, or other mechanical, chemical, or psychic irritations. "Once produced," claims the association, "the lesion becomes a focus of sustained pathological irritation."

While Palmer's theory of disease has been modified, the primary chiropractic treatment for all human illness remains the same as in 1895: spinal adjustment.

Chiropractic adjustment is a specific form of spinal manipulation. The technique, which is also used occasionally by osteopaths, physical therapists, and some medical doctors, is distinguished by the suddenness or speed of the maneuver, which prevents any control by the patient. By comparison, a patient can voluntarily resist—and therefore control—a manipulation when the therapist does it slowly or rythmically. If there is pain, for example, the patient can physically prevent further movement or advise the therapist accordingly. The latter technique, which is generally called *mobilization*, is the most common type of joint manipulation used by physical therapists.

In contrast, chiropractors emphasize the sudden maneuver, which they call a *dynamic thrust*. It may be done gently or forcefully, but always with a quick movement. The maneuver often produces a click-like sound in the manipulated joint.

Those medical and osteopathic practitioners who use this technique say that it is sometimes effective for treating certain joint abnormalities or pain originating in the back or neck. There is disagreement among them, however, about what conditions it helps and exactly how it does so.

One prominent theory is that the manipulation essentially restores joint mobility, including a measure of "joint play" that isn't apparent in voluntary movements. Another is that the technique may displace a small fragment of a spinal disk that may be pressing against adjacent tissue. Others suggest that the sudden force may stretch a contracted muscle or tear adhesions, possibly relieving a local pain-causing spasm. Some manipulators subscribe to one theory while others believe several are possible. As yet, there's no proof that any of these theories are correct.

The chiropractic explanation is that the maneuver corrects subluxations. The current chiropractic definition of subluxation is so broad, however, that it takes in virtually any mechanical or functional derangement of the spine— or, as one speaker at the NIH workshop put it, "any variance from the normalcy of a newborn child." As a result, the chiropractic view does not reject any of the other theories. A locked joint or offending disk fragment would simply be labeled a subluxation.

Thus, most manipulators believe that their action affects some local condition, whatever it may be. The real quarrel arises when chiropractors claim that their manipulation *also* influences the nervous system and helps prevent or cure disease, an issue we will discuss later in this report.

Despite chiropractic's origin and all-embracing theory of disease, many persons tend to view chiropractors as specialists in muscle or joint problems, particularly those of the back.

Part of the reason, of course, is that chiropractic manipulation focuses on the spine. Whatever its ultimate intent, the therapy involves direct, physical action on the back. So people may conclude that that's what the treatment is for.

But there are other reasons as well for this traditional association. For one thing, the medical contemporary of the early chiropractor gave little priority to back ailments. The new science of bacteriology held immense promise for treating otherwise fatal illnesses, as did other developments in diagnosis and surgery. Hence, medical efforts in the first third of this century focused on infectious disease and similarly urgent problems. Backaches could wait. Not until the 1930s did the medical profession start paying much attention to physical medicine and rehabilitation. In the interim, chiropractic seemed to offer hope in an area that medicine had largely ignored.

Even today, many physicians find little satisfaction in treating back ailments. Chronic pain may often be influenced by psychological problems or physical habits that patients are unable or unwilling to change. Exact diagnosis can be elusive and expensive, and follow-up treatment can be time-consuming for the doctor. Specialists in physical medicine and orthopedics interviewed by CU asserted that, too often, treatment by some physicians simply meant prescribing a painkiller, muscle relaxant, or tranquilizer rather than taking the time and effort such ailments might demand.

Chiropractors, meanwhile, have usually been ready and willing to see patients repeatedly and provide active treatment—manipulation, exercise programs, heat application, and the like. In CU's opinion, such accommodation has probably reinforced the belief that chiropractors specialize in back ailments. Indeed, a survey conducted several years ago by the University of Kentucky College of Medicine revealed that most of the people in the study who visited chiropractors believed that a chiropractor has more specialized training in musculoskeletal back and joint problems than a physician has. Actually, chiropractors usually have more training than medical doctors in only one area: manipulative therapy.

Chiropractors who belong to the International Chiropractors Association (about 37 percent of practitioners) often confine their treatment solely to manipulation. Besides spinal adjustment, treatment may include various "soft-tissue" manipulations, such as massaging muscles or applying sustained pressure to ligaments. But the basic approach is "hands only."

Most other chiropractors, however, use a variety of treatment techniques. The scope generally depends on what's permitted by state or provincial law. Chiropractors may not practice surgery or order prescription drugs. But many jurisdictions allow them to use physiotherapy and to recommend various nutritional supplements, such as vitamins and minerals.

The types of treatment are often similar to some used by physicians or physical therapists (although the purpose of application may not always be the same). In addition to exercise programs, such measures may include the use of braces or casts, whirlpool baths, hot or cold packs, ultrasound, diathermy machines, and other devices.

Chiropractic, in short, is seldom limited to spinal adjustment alone. Chiropractors often can, and do, make use of common measures for treating muscle or joint complaints. And some limit their practice almost exclusively to such complaints, frankly dismissing Palmer's disease theory as "cultism" or "chiroquackery."

An undetermined number also try to cooperate with local physicians, referring to them patients who appear to need medical care and occasionally receiving a referral in turn. In April 1975, for instance, *Medical Economics*, a magazine distributed to physicians, reported the response of more than a thousand office-based MDs to a survey it conducted of referral relationships with chiropractors. More than 20 percent stated that they received some referrals from chiropractors. Also 5 percent of the respondents said they sometimes referred patients to chiropractors.

On the basis of CU's investigation, however, such instances of cooperation, or of chiropractic willingness to limit its scope of practice, tend to be the exception rather than the rule. Chiropractic officials and educators invariably told CU that the chiropractor's role was that of a *pri-*

mary physician, not a muscle-and-joint practitioner. They emphasized that chiropractors should serve as one of the "portals of entry" to the health-care system, functioning essentially as family doctors and referring patients, when appropriate, to other health professions.

Such a role assumes that chiropractors, despite much less diagnostic training than MDs or DOs, will recognize when to treat a patient and when to refer one to a physician. It's on this point—and on the question of scientific validity—that chiropractic clashes most seriously with organized medicine.

For years, chiropractic spokesmen have argued that medical or scientific opposition to chiropractic is largely a business quarrel. According to the charge, organized medicine is a monopoly concerned primarily with aggrandizement of physicians, and the American Medical Association (AMA) is just trying to keep out the competition. The book *Chiropractic: A Modern Way to Health,* which was recommended to CU by chiropractic officials, typically points the accusing finger at the AMA: ". . . the AMA is a private group of men and women with a common private business interest, namely the practice of medicine," writes the author, Julius Dintenfass, DC, a charter member of the New York State Board of Chiropractic Examiners. "Despite their vaunted concern for the public health and welfare, the medical sachems act toward chiropractic as any collection of businessmen being threatened by a rival concern which seems to have the kind of merchandise that customers prefer."

When CU discussed the allegation with chiropractic officials, we expected to find wide agreement with it. We didn't.

"It's not true," said Richard C. Schafer, DC, director of public affairs for the ACA, in an interview with CU. "The average medical doctor has more patients than he can handle," Dr. Schafer said. "They're not afraid of competition."

Why, then, does organized medicine oppose chiropractic?

CU got several answers from AMA representatives and other critics. They involved charges of inferior education and training, rejection of medical science, and abuses or hazards arising from the practice of chiropractic.

Since those allegations have serious implications for patient care and safety, CU investigated them in detail.

There is virtually no denial that educational standards for chiropractors in the past were often little short of appalling. As late as 1942, according to *Medical Economics*, it was still possible to get the mail-order Doctor of Chiropractic degree from a Chicago college for $127.50.

Although standards later improved, glaring deficiencies prevailed until recent years. The scope of the problem was outlined in a thorough evaluation of chiropractic schools conducted in 1964 by Dewey Anderson, PhD, who was at that time the director of education for the ACA. Some of the inadequacies that were mentioned in Dr. Anderson's 1964 report were: "Too many instructors teaching the basic sciences without having had any advanced or graduate training in these sciences. Too many instructors not trained or qualified as teachers nor masters of their fields, resulting in slavish devotion to textbook teaching and instruction considerably below the level of post-college professional education."

The academic credentials of the students, Dr. Anderson noted, were similarly deficient: "One of the most serious handicaps . . . is that of trying to teach at the post-college professional level students who for the most part have not gone beyond high school, and who in high school were not in the upper half of their classes. For many of them a professional college course is too difficult to master."

The result, said Dr. Anderson, was to downgrade instruction so that students could pass the courses.

A comprehensive study of chiropractic conducted in 1965 for the government of Quebec reached similar conclusions. Student admission requirements were termed "too liberal, and inadequate," and the training required of teachers was judged "definitely inferior" to that demanded either by medical schools or by university science departments. "A great number of these teachers are chiropractors who have received training in basic sciences of very little value," said the Quebec study.

Landmark studies of chiropractic by the United States Department of Health, Education, and Welfare (HEW) in 1968 and Ontario's Committee on the Healing Arts in 1970 expressed similarly critical findings. In addition to poorly qualified teachers, inferior basic science courses, and notably low admission requirements, both reports criticized the lack of emphasis on research. The HEW report also noted the absence of inpatient hospital training and a poor ratio of faculty to students. At the time of HEW's study, chiropractic schools averaged about one faculty member for each nineteen students, compared with 1 per 1.7 students in medical schools. (Both figures include part-time instructors with administrative duties or outside practices.)

"The scope and quality of chiropractic education do not prepare the practitioner to make an adequate diagnosis and provide appropriate treatment," the HEW report concluded. The Ontario committee endorsed HEW's findings on education and judged the chiropractor's diagnostic ability as "very limited at best."

A study conducted for the state of Wisconsin in 1972 found conditions largely unchanged. While commending the "sincerity and dedication" of both students and faculty, the Wisconsin study committee concluded that "the deficiencies are too pervasive to permit an adequate educational experience."

Since the early 1970s, chiropractic schools have actively sought to raise their educational standards. This was evident at the colleges CU visited. They still require only a "C" average for admission, but entering students must now have two years of college or the equivalent, including courses in biology and chemistry. Actually, about half of the current entrants at National College of Chiropractic in Lombard, Ill., and at Canadian Memorial College of Chiropractic in Toronto already have college degrees.

The change in the academic background of students is perhaps most dramatic at Palmer College of Chiropractic in Davenport, Iowa, which is by far the world's largest chiropractic school (Palmer trains about one-third of all chiropractors). Its January 1975 enrollment still included about 550 students whose previous education was limited to high school or an equivalency program. Virtually all were seniors scheduled to graduate that year, however. The rest of Palmer's 2,100 students had one or more years of college; 416 of them held college degrees.

Academic requirements for faculty members have also been upgraded. Increasingly, instructors in basic science subjects must have recognized qualifications in their disciplines, and the colleges are giving preference to candidates with graduate degrees.

Insistence on advanced qualifications tends to be most pronounced at National College. Instructors in basic sciences must generally have a graduate degree in their specialty, and the college says it will not hire a teacher with only a master's degree unless the candidate's department already includes a PhD. A DC degree is still acceptable, though, for instructors in chiropractic or clinical courses.

In short, chiropractors are no longer teaching all subjects. And the colleges have also narrowed the ratio of faculty to students. Canadian Memorial, for example, has roughly one teacher for every eight students. Instructors are still spread fairly thin at Palmer, with one per thirty students. But that's an improvement over its 1-to-45 ratio of a few years ago. Library facilities have also been expanded, and National College, for one, has initiated a modest research project with a federal agency.

Despite improvements in other areas, education in diagnosis remains a stepchild—especially in comparison with training received by physicians. Part of the problem is historical. Traditionally, chiropractors believed it wasn't important to "name" a disease. The important thing was to find and correct the subluxation allegedly causing it. It made little difference, for example, if a liver disorder involved congestion, cirrhosis, or cancer; the object was to relieve nervous-system disturbances that were supposedly responsible for the disorder.

Accordingly, that approach placed little or no emphasis on making a *differential* diagnosis—that is, one that considers possible causes of a patient's symptoms and establishes probable as well as alternative diagnoses. While differential diagnosis is fundamental in the practice of medicine, chiropractors generally shunned it, preferring to call their approach "spinal analysis" rather than diagnosis. Even today, some practitioners insist that medical diagnosis is out of place in chiropractic.

"It is a trap for the unwary in this profession," wrote William D. Harper, DC, president of Texas Chiropractic College, in 1975 in *The Digest of Chiropractic Economics*. "We waste too much time in our curriculum on medical diagnosis."

Many chiropractic officials and educators disagree with

that sentiment, however. And diagnostic training is now an integral part of the curriculum at most chiropractic colleges. Yet most of the people *teaching* diagnosis are the very same chiropractors who were trained in the 1960s and earlier, when educational standards—and attitudes toward diagnosis—were far from ideal. Those instructors, moreover, labor under a burden common to all chiropractors—the lack of inpatient hospital training.

"The medical doctor has the benefit of patient exposure that we do not have," says Andries M. Kleynhans, DC, director of clinical sciences at National College. Because of the lack of chiropractic hospitals, chiropractors seldom see or treat diseases that the medical doctor does. That gap, Dr. Kleynhans told CU, places chiropractors at a disadvantage in their diagnostic training.

In addition, chiropractors cannot use many of the sophisticated diagnostic techniques available to the physician. This is true even for some major diagnostic aids involving the spine. A herniated spinal disk, for example, isn't visible on a simple X-ray. If it's necessary to confirm the disk protrusion, a physician may order a myelogram, an X-ray technique that involves injecting an opaque dye into the space surrounding the spinal cord. Chiropractors are neither trained to interpret myelograms nor permitted to perform them.

Nor do they have the benefit of the more extensive education and training required of physicians. In contrast to the chiropractor's two years of college (now) and four years of professional school, the physician must have four years of college, four years of medical school, and usually three or more years of hospital residency. Moreover, the physician's subsequent affiliation with a hospital provides a center for continuing education. At the hospital, the physician's medical knowledge is reinforced and expanded through conferences, discussions, and association with colleagues, as well as through experiences with patients. Chiropractors, in comparison, generally work alone.

Clearly, the scope, quality, and length of chiropractic education cannot provide the depth of diagnostic training a physician receives. Even more fundamental, however, is the validity of what the chiropractor learns. If it's unsound, more training might only compound the error. The crucial question, therefore, is whether chiropractic theory is true or false.

The belief that minor interference with the spinal nerves can cause or aggravate disease is the cornerstone of chiropractic theory. It is also the focus of scientific objections. A few anatomical facts may help to explain why.

There are twenty-six pairs of nerves that exit from mobile segments of the spine. They are the only part of the nervous system conceivably accessible to manipulation. Twelve pairs of cranial nerves, which exit through openings in the base of the skull and bypass the spine, are out of reach of manipulation. So, too, are five pairs exiting from the sacrum, a solid bone formed by the fusion of five vertebrae in the lower spine. The spinal cord (which is surrounded by spinal fluid as well as by protective layers of tissue) and the brain itself—with all its interconnecting nerve pathways—are also out of reach.

Thus, the chiropractor's action is exerted on only a limited part of the nervous system. It excludes, for example, the nerves of sight, hearing, taste, and smell, and the entire parasympathetic nervous system. The latter, along with the sympathetic nervous system, form the balancing halves of the autonomic, or "involuntary," nervous system, which serves the vital organs.

Scientists, of course, accept the importance of the nervous system in body functions. What they reject, however, is the assertion that manipulation directed at a limited part of this intricate system can prevent or cure disease. In the first place, there's no scientific evidence that minor off-centerings of the vertebrae impinge on spinal nerves. One study in 1973, which tested fresh cadaver spines, suggested that impingement does not occur even when the spine is twisted into extreme positions or abnormal forces are applied to the vertebrae. Second, if such a partial block could occur, its effect would be nil. Research by neurophysiologists shows that a nerve impulse travels more slowly in a zone of partial compression but resumes its flow immediately thereafter. The impulse transmitted is normal in all respects. What is perhaps hardest for scientists to accept, though, is chiropractic's singular concept of the nervous system itself.

According to that view, the nervous system is the overall master of all body functions, regulating everything from major organs to intricate cellular activities. A typical statement of this concept appears in the current pamphlet, *How Chiropractic Heals,* one of many such pamphlets for patients distributed by chiropractors. "None of the body functions 'just happen,'" says the pamphlet. "Your heart doesn't just happen to beat. Your lungs don't just happen to inhale and exhale. Your stomach doesn't just happen to digest your dinner. *All* doctors know that your brain and nerve system coordinate these functions which make for life instead of death, health instead of sickness."

Actually, all doctors know no such thing. The heart just *does* happen to beat. It will beat for a period of time even if removed from the body and cut off from all nerve impulses, so long as it's surrounded by a nutrient fluid. Transplanted, it is capable of sustaining life in another human being without any immediate connection to the brain, spinal cord, or other nerve tissue. The heart has an intrinsic rhythm of its own and thus can function automatically.

Similarly, the stomach digests automatically. There are *inherent* processes that govern the functions of organs as important as the heart, stomach, intestines, blood vessels, and the like. Their function doesn't depend entirely on the nervous system. A paraplegic woman, for example, may conceive, carry her pregnancy to term, and give birth to a normal baby—despite severe injury to her spinal cord. Except for bladder and bowel problems, internal organs of a quadriplegic still continue to function, even though the spinal nerves are useless from the neck down. In short, life goes on—despite even massive "interference" with nerve impulses. That doesn't mean the spinal nerves aren't important. But their importance doesn't render other fundamental life processes trivial.

The immunological defense system, for instance, can work independently of nerve impulses. Artificially cultured white blood cells will continue to engulf germs even though entirely divorced from nerve influence. At the cellular level, to which chiropractic claims to extend, the same autonomy has been documented. Molecular research has become so precise that it can sometimes pinpoint which portion of a molecule is responsible for a particular disease. These biochemical life processes are fundamental—and completely independent of the nervous system.

Not a single scientific study in the eighty-year existence of chiropractic or the entire history of medicine shows that manipulation can affect any of these basic life processes. But a vast amount of evidence suggests it cannot.

In 1895, neither Palmer nor his contemporaries could foresee that research. Today, however, there's no excuse for ignoring it. Unless most medical research in the twentieth century is wrong, Palmer's disease theory belongs in the pages of nineteenth-century history, with bleeding, purging, and other blind alleys of medicine.

When chiropractic theory is put into practice, its efforts can sometimes border on the ludicrous. Several chiropractic pamphlets that have been used in Canada, for example, tout spinal manipulation as a cure for childhood bed-wetting. Actually, the nerves to the bladder emerge from the rigid bone of the sacrum. There is no way to manipulate them. Further, a true nerve defect would cause constant bladder problems, not just bed-wetting.

Spinal manipulation is also promoted frequently for patients with high blood pressure. A typical pamphlet obtained from the sales department at Palmer College suggests that the ailment may be treated through "proper adjustment by hand."

While the basic causes of high blood pressure in most patients are still unknown, the portion of the nervous system involved in lowering blood pressure is well identified—the parasympathetic nervous system. It is fed by the cranial and sacral nerves, and, as noted earlier, is entirely inaccessible to manipulation.

Another pamphlet from Palmer, entitled *Eye Trouble*, suggests that manipulation may be applicable to some eye problems. The optic nerves are completely self-contained in the skull. There is no conceivable way to reach them manually.

Other pamphlets obtained from Palmer tout manipulation for conditions ranging from acne and appendicitis to stomach trouble and tonsillitis. There isn't a shred of scientific evidence showing that those ailments respond to manipulation.

Such unproved claims have bedeviled some chiropractors for years. In an August 1974 letter, Herbert W. E. Poinsett, a Florida chiropractor, took the ACA to task for one of its pamphlets. "The new ACA tract on the kidneys is a disgrace to this profession," wrote Dr. Poinsett. "The statement, 'Your doctor of chiropractic treats many kidney disorders,' is pure nonsense! I ask you, what disorders?

"Does chiropractic treat the following successfully? Neoplasms, tumors of the adrenal gland, calculi, hydronephrosis, tuberculosis, nonspecific infections. . . .

"Are you telling the people that we can treat such pathologies? If you are, then we deserve the title of quack and cultists!"

"Many within the profession, I'm sure, may agree with your comments," an ACA official replied. However, he noted, others might want to utilize the tract in their practices. "This tract, in one version or another, has been a stock item for over forty years and has been redesigned to meet the sustained needs of the interested membership."

Most chiropractic officials interviewed by CU frankly admitted the problem of over-claiming. "We as a profession have claimed too much without valid proof," said Donald C. Sutherland, DC, executive director of the Canadian Chiropractic Association. He indicated that the Canadian organization was actively trying to limit chiropractic's scope of practice. Neither in Canada nor in the United States, however, could CU find concrete evidence that abuses in the field were abating.

At the Sherman College of Chiropractic in Spartanburg, S.C., for example, the criteria for accepting a patient are liberal indeed. According to an editorial by Douglas Gates, a dean of the college, requirements for a "chiropractic case" are threefold: Does the patient have a spinal column? Does the patient have a nervous system? Is the patient alive?

For some chiropractors, economics probably plays a large part in the range of illnesses treated. A limited scope of practice can often mean fewer patients. And those who confine themselves to musculoskeletal problems—sprains, strains, and back or neck ailments—tend to cut their income potential.

According to the ACA, United States chiropractors in 1974 earned an average annual income of about $31,000. Canadian practitioners averaged roughly the same. Often contributing to the attainment of that income are various practice-building organizations that seem to abound within the profession.

Among the oldest of such groups is the Parker Chiropractic Research Foundation, which offers a comprehensive, hard-sell approach for attracting patients and keeping them coming back. Over the last twenty years, several thousand chiropractors or their assistants have attended the Parker courses.

Parker encourages practitioners to advertise and stresses the use of a Chiropractic Research Chart and a "nerve" chart. The former lists numerous disorders purportedly helped by chiropractic treatment and gives the percentage of "success" for each. The nerve chart shows a picture of the spine and specifies the diseases supposedly caused by misalignments at each level.

Neither chart has any scientific validity or any acceptable evidence to support its claims. Because of such advertising, the Canadian Chiropractic Association refuses to release its mailing list to the Parker organization.

Another of the most successful practice builders is Clinic Masters, which claims a membership of about 12 percent of all United States and Canadian chiropractors in active practice. According to its membership contract, a chiropractor who "desires to have the Clinic Masters System revealed to him" must agree to pay $10,000 and not "divulge or share, directly or indirectly," any portion of the system with anyone other than a Clinic Masters client.

Clinic Masters teaches a variety of specific income-building techniques and promotes the idea that higher income means greater service to patients. Some ways of providing such service includes multiple billing, which means charging for *each* spinal adjustment or other unit of treatment rather than accepting a flat office fee; a "case basis" approach, which involves charging by the case (like a surgeon) rather than by number of visits; and "intensive day care," which adds room or ward fees to the bill.

In recognition of their "service to humanity," clients earn membership ranks in one of twelve Clinic Masters clubs. The lowest is the Leviathan club, for those earning $4,000 to $8,000 a month. The highest is the Purple & White Medallion club, which was recently added for members earning $50,000 or more a month.

According to the major chiropractic associations, none of the billing practices mentioned above is considered "a reasonable and customary procedure" in the profession. But criticism has been stifled somewhat by Clinic Masters' threat to sue those whose remarks it judges to be libelous. It offers a $10,000 reward to anyone who is first to report and substantiate "disparaging statements about Clinic Masters" that lead to a successful lawsuit.

Despite the excesses of some practitioners and chiropractic's rejection of science, the profession nevertheless maintains that it offers an important health service. And each year more than five million men, women, and children obtain chiropractic treatment in the United States and Canada. Many of those patients sincerely believe that chiropractors help them, that those practitioners are a good deal more than common quacks. In fact, how may patients sometimes benefit from chiropractic treatment? And what risks do they face in the process?

HOW CHIROPRACTORS CAN HELP—OR HARM

Years ago some surgeons thought they had developed a promising cure for angina, the chest pains associated with coronary heart disease. Tying off an artery in the chest appeared to offer relief. The cure was short-lived, however. Subsequent research showed that a sham operation, consisting of just a superficial incision on the chest wall, was equally successful.

That experiment, like countless others, demonstrated the broad influence of the "placebo-effect," a psychological reaction to a medication or procedure that results in improvement or cure of symptoms. Because of it, a sham operation may ease anginal pain or a dummy pill may relieve the nausea of pregnancy.

It matters little whether the treatment is surgery, drugs, manipulation, or incantations. The key factors in the placebo effect are the patient's confidence in the healer and the healer's faith in the therapy—especially when that faith is communicated to the patient.

Throughout much of medical history, the placebo effect was frequently all any healer could offer. Indeed, a patient was often fortunate if the actual treatment was of psychological value, or even merely worthless, rather than harmful or fatal. Today, despite all the acumen and paraphernalia of modern medicine, such psychological effects are still an important factor in therapy. And they frequently account for some of the benefits obtained from the most skilled of physicians. They also explain, in part, why chiropractors can sometimes help people.

Physicians have long recognized the potent psychological effect of the "laying on of hands." Chiropractors at the NIH conference in February 1975 also acknowledged its role in treatment. In fact, one prominent chiropractic speaker, Dr. Scott Haldeman of Vancouver, B.C., felt that such placebo effects should be considered an advantage of manipulation.

"Clinicians who practice spinal manipulations often become very defensive when their detractors derisively state that all results can be explained on the basis of psychological effects," Dr. Haldeman said. "However, there are very few therapies that have the advantages of laying on of hands, relaxing tense muscles, causing a sensation in the area of pain, the click or pop of the adjustment, and a clinician who has complete confidence in his therapy. It is a pity that this possibility has been considered a criticism of the therapeutic procedure instead of one of its advantages."

Numerous studies show that placebo treatment in many disorders helps about one-third of patients. Temporary relief of pain or other symptoms has been demonstrated, for example, in arthritis, hay fever, headache, cough, high blood pressure, peptic ulcer, and even cancer.

The psychological aspects of many disorders also work to the healer's advantage. According to CU's interviews with specialists in internal medicine, one-third to one-half of the complaints patients present in routine office visits either have obvious psychological origins or do not arise from organic disease. Hence, treatment offering some psychological benefit can often be helpful. A sympathetic ear for the patient's complaints or firm, authoritative reassurance that no serious disease is involved can prove therapeutic in itself.

One of the most important factors, suggested a physician at the NIH conference, is that patients are relieved of the responsibility of their illness and suffering when they hand that burden over to the healer. "That silent act," he asserted, "is probably . . . as important as anything else that goes on, and often many of the things that we do after that point we get by with rather than being effective with."

Beyond psychological influences in treatment, there are also the recuperative powers of the body itself. Medical scientists estimate that about two-thirds of human illness is self-limiting. Regardless of what type of outside intervention or treatment is used, the patients eventually get well by themselves.

"If it were more than that figure . . . I suspect there'd be no need for any of us." commented Fletcher McDowell, MD, of Cornell University, to the NIH conference participants. "If it were less than 50 percent, we'd either all be out of work or in jail, I'm not sure which."

Even some chronic disorders, such as rheumatoid arthritis or multiple sclerosis, have spontaneous remissions. The symptoms may disappear, regardless of treatment, for months or more, affording temporary or, at times, long-term relief. If the patient happens to be under treatment at the time, the practitioner and the type of therapy may get credit for such relief.

Most back problems will also resolve themselves. Several studies show that about 60 percent of patients with back pain get well within three weeks and at least 90 percent recover within two months—regardless of the type of treatment received. Only about 2 percent eventually undergo surgery, usually for serious bone or disk problems.

Although physicians and chiropractors emphasize different methods of treatment in common back problems, a recent study comparing both groups showed essentially no difference in the outcome of therapy. Both the physicians and the chiropractors achieved satisfactory results with more than 90 percent of patients suffering from back or neck ailments.

Perhaps the most interesting part of the study, which was conducted by researchers at the University of Utah College of Medicine, was the reaction of patients to their respective practitioners. The chiropractic patients were significantly more satisfied with the explanations they received about their problems and the degree to which they were made to feel welcome.

Reporting their findings in *The Lancet*, a British medical journal, in June 1974, the authors stressed the implications of the patients' reactions: "On the basis of our study and others, it appears that the chiropractor may be more attuned to the total needs of the patient than is his medical counterpart. The chiropractor does not seem hurried. He uses language patients can understand. He gives them sympathy, and he is patient with them. He does not take a superior attitude toward them. In summary, it is an egalitarian relationship rather than a superordinate/subordinate relationship."

Their findings, the authors concluded, "underscore the powerful potential for the doctor-patient relationship in effective treatment, whether in chiropractic or traditional medicine."

Many positive responses to chiropractic treatment undoubtedly stem from the doctor-patient relationship or the self-limiting nature of various illnesses. But some favorable results can be ascribed directly to manipulation itself.

Government studies in the United States and Canada have judged manipulation to be a potentially useful technique for certain conditions, such as the loss of joint mobility. Research in manipulation is still meager, and controlled clinical studies are rare. But chiropractors and other practitioners who use manipulative therapy agree it can help some muscle or joint problems.

Treatment of tension headaches by massage, for example, is well recognized. Those headaches can stem from tense muscles in the neck, and proper massage may relieve symptoms. Some practitioners also report that a stiff joint in the neck may sometimes cause headache pain that can be treated by manipulation.

In general, back or neck pain that might arise from restricted movement in a spinal joint may respond to manipulation. Such pain is usually localized in the area of the joint. The pain may sometimes be referred to another part of the body, such as the chest, however. Such referred pain may occasionally mimic the symptoms of other disorders, such as angina.

"Thus we find a perfectly reasonable basis in fact for the somewhat bizarre stories of miraculous cures by spinal manipulation," says John McM. Mennell, MD, an authority on manipulative therapy. "Almost invariably the basis of these stories is that the patient has been told a diagnosis which he believes and remembers," writes Dr. Mennell in his book, *Back Pain*. "If his symptoms are then unrelieved by orthodox treatment, but are later cured by a manipulator, it is not surprising that the patient claims to have been cured of the visceral disease." Many chiropractors and other manipulators share Dr. Mennell's view.

There are, in short, a variety of possible reasons why patients may experience benefits from chiropractic treatment. That may not be all they experience, however. The Chiropractic Study Committee for the State of Wisconsin in 1972 underscored a critical issue surrounding chiropractic: "It is beyond question that substantial numbers of people believe themselves to have been helped by chiropractic treatment," said the committee report. "It is also beyond question that if they feel better, for whatever reason, they have, in some sense, been helped. There is, however, a balancing factor that screams to be considered. That, of course, is the potential hazard of treatment that ignores established scientific knowledge."

On the basis of CU's investigation, there are several major areas for concern. Since many human illnesses are self-resolving, any intervention by a practitioner should avoid exposing a patient to unnecessary risks. The maxim, as a medical aphorism puts it, is *primum non nocere*: "First of all, do no harm."

The ACA states that spinal manipulation is "a painless and safe procedure." But a review of chiropractic and medical literature by CU indicates that manipulation is not without hazard. The adverse effects reported range from minor sprains and soreness to serious complications and death. Serious complications included fracture, spinal disk rupture, paraplegia, and stroke. Chiropractors say that such catastrophic consequences of manipulation as stroke are relatively rare; and, indeed, CU's investigation uncovered only twelve documented cases of severe stroke from chiropractic manipulation since 1947.

The exact incidence of injury is virtually impossible to determine, however. Unlike medical reports, none of the many chiropractic surveys or journals that CU reviewed gave any statistics on complication. The only data are from isolated medical studies by a few physicians.

In an attempt to fill that gap, a study published in *Clinical Orthopaedics and Related Research* in 1971 reported the injuries from chiropractic manipulation recorded by one physician over a three-year period. The physician reported that 172 of the patients he examined in his practice had previously undergone chiropractic manipulation. Seven of those, or 4 percent, had suffered direct injuries, ranging from aggravation of pain to serious nerve damage. "Injury associated with spinal manipulation," the physician concluded, "appears more frequent than the present North

American medical literature suggests."

Therapy often involves risks. The question is whether those risks are warranted. Many surgical procedures and drugs used in medical practice are hazardous. Accordingly, physicians will weigh such risks against the proven value of treatment so that patients will not be endangered unnecessarily. While an individual physician's judgment may be faulty, the emphasis of medicine on proven therapy tends to increase the average patient's chances of genuine therapeutic benefits for the risks taken.

If spinal manipulation were a proven form of universal therapy, there would be no reason to restrict it to muscle or joint disorders, even if it involved some risk. But as CU pointed out in the first part of this report, chiropractic use of manipulation in other illnesses contradicts much of the basic medical research of the twentieth century. In such applications, CU concludes, any risk of injury is unwarranted.

Unlike physicians, chiropractors receive no education or training in pharmacology or drug therapy. What they learn about drugs is often self-taught. That lack of scientific background or experience in drug therapy may well contribute to what CU views as a dangerous approach to drugs by many chiropractors. Specifically, it involves undermining the use of accepted drug therapies and espousing the use of unproven ones.

Various chiropractic pamphlets for the public employ direct scare tactics against drugs. Such titles as *Drug-Caused Diseases* and *Drugs—Dangerous Whether Pushed or Prescribed* are typical. One published by the ACA, *Beware of Overuse of Drugs*, lists scores of possible adverse reactions to such drugs as antibiotics, oral contraceptives, and medicines for high blood pressure. The pamphlet then asserts that chiropractors use no drugs, "thus avoiding drug-induced illnesses and dangerous side effects often more serious than the condition being treated." There's no mention that some of those drugs may be life-saving for patients who need them.

A common tactic is to link drug-taking with drug-abuse. "Don't be a pill popper," says the headline of an ad put out by the ACA. "Drugging your pain and your problems is not your answer to good health." According to the ad, "drugs and medications only mask the pain and dull the symptoms of a health problem."

The consequences of such advice can be tragic. These are typical of the cases CU has come across:

■ Under chiropractic care, an elderly woman with high blood pressure was advised to stop medication. Her blood pressure rose sharply, and after a month she suffered a stroke.

■ A diabetic patient gave up insulin on instruction of a chiropractor. An infection held in check by good control of the diabetes with insulin then spread and caused the patient's death.

■ Parents of a six-year-old epileptic girl stopped anticonvulsive therapy on the advice of a chiropractor. Until then, the child had been doing well and was seizure-free. Without the medication, she had a prolonged seizure that resulted in brain damage and subsequent mental retardation.

Chiropractic antipathy to medication, however, appears limited to *prescription* drugs—which chiropractors may not legally order. Other medications, such as vitamin preparations, are widely recommended and sold in chiropractic practice. In CU's opinion, that distinction can be a dangerous one. A substance is defined as a drug by its use, not by arbitrary categories. In medicine, a drug is any substance used as medication for a disease. Water prescribed for a dehydrated patient can be defined as a drug. Ordering vitamins for a deficiency disease is prescribing a drug.

For the patient's safety, any prescriber should have sufficient training to know when and why a specific drug is indicated. Chiropractors have no such training. In CU's view, a brief course in nutrition at a chiropractic school is no substitute for years of training in drug therapy. Yet chiropractors sometimes presume they can treat complex illnesses with vitamin pills.

An article in the March 1975 issue of *The ACA Journal of Chiropractic*, for example, espoused high-dose vitamins for treating schizophrenia, a complex and sometimes crippling mental illness. The author noted that "there is a great deal of controversy" surrounding such treatment, but he concluded that "the megavitamin approach is a practical alternative" for treating schizophrenia. The approach, he said, "should be considered by chiropractic as an adjunct to spinal manipulation."

Indeed, there once was "a great deal of controversy" about megavitamin therapy for schizophrenia. But that was before several carefully controlled studies showed it to have no therapeutic benefit. On the contrary, the findings suggested potentially adverse effects, including longer hospitalization, increased need for other drugs, and poorer adjustment to home and community life after patients left the hospital. Overall, the treatment was judged inferior to a placebo. Thus, the chiropractic author is recommending that a complicated mental disorder be treated with a drug less effective than a dummy pill.

One of the worst dangers of chiropractic treatment, say its critics, is that it might divert the patient from seeking appropriate medical attention in time. The result, they contend, may have serious or even fatal consequences that might otherwise have been avoided.

Part of the problem is the confusing nature of back pain.

Most patients who visit chiropractors go initially because of back troubles. But back pain can arise from a variety of conditions, from a simple sprain to heart disease. It may be muscular or skeletal in origin, or a symptom of ulcers, cancer, or disorders of the uterus or ovaries. It can also be caused by diseases of the lungs, kidneys, liver, bladder, intestines, or other organs.

When a disorder of the internal organs is suspected, many chiropractors will refer the patient to a physician. But the chiropractor's limited diagnostic training presents a major handicap to early recognition of such illnesses. And some chiropractors will continue to treat a patient regardless of any diagnosis, apparently convinced by chiropractic theory that they are relieving the true cause of the disease. Meanwhile, the illness may grow worse.

There is relatively little information available about the type or frequency of serious consequences resulting from such delays. According to AMA officials, physicians are usually reluctant to report such instances for fear of lawsuits. The court cases that CU is aware of, however, show that delays in proper treatment have resulted in mental retardation, paralysis, and deaths from tuberculosis, spinal meningitis, and cancer.

In most of those cases, the victims were young children. The most bitter criticism of chiropractic that CU encountered, in fact, was from pediatric hospitals. Some of the reasons why were underscored in a report issued jointly in 1972 by the Montreal Children's Hospital and the St. Justine Hospital for Children.

The report described pamphlets distributed by chiropractors to patients in Quebec. The pamphlets claimed that chiropractors could treat epilepsy, croup, cross-eye, rheumatic fever, bronchitis, pneumonia, appendicitis, leukemia, and other illnesses affecting children. Such claims, said the report, constituted "a real and direct danger" to children. "This is especially so in that many childhood illnesses are of an acute nature and require diagnosis and treatment without delay."

For example, one pamphlet then in circulation entitled *Chiropractic for Children,* advised spinal manipulation for croup. "In actual fact," said the report of the children's hospitals, "croup is an acute infectious disease involving the voice-box area of the throat. It often requires prompt medical attention which at times may be lifesaving." Cross-eye, too, should be treated at a relatively early age, or blindness may result in the affected eye, said the report.

Parents faced with a desperate situation, such as a child with leukemia, need balanced and mature advice, the report stressed. "By calling himself a 'doctor,' by taking X-Rays, by pretending to be qualified, the chiropractor creates a false image as to his ability to deal with pediatric problems. This leads directly to delay in the proper diagnosis being made and the correct therapy being started, which might affect the child for the rest of his life."

The report also decried earlier opposition of chiropractic authorities to immunization. If those princples had been accepted, said the report, "then this world would now be filled with smallpox, people paralyzed [or] dead from tetanus, children choking to death from diphtheria, the uncontrolled spread of typhoid . . . and innocent children living in iron lungs because of polio."

According to a survey conducted by the ACA in August 1973, about 81 percent of its members reported that they treat children. Those chiropractors saw an average of ninety-three children annually, about 30 percent of whom were of preschool age. Respiratory ailments, allergies, and nervous-system disorders were among the five most frequently treated conditions.

Each of the major chiropractic associations in the United States and Canada publishes pamphlets promoting chiropractic care for children. None of the current ones that CU reviewed makes claims about treating infectious diseases, nor do they argue against immunization of children. But the alarm expressed in 1972 by the two Canadian children's hospitals appears to us to be no less justified today.

Of particular concern, in our view, is advice published in the October 1974 issue of *The ACA Journal of Chiropractic*. An article entitled "Pediatrics" recommended chiropractic treatment for children with infectious diseases, digestive disorders, respiratory illnesses, heart problems, genitourinary disorders, and other illnesses. "The infectious diseases usually respond well to chiropractic care," said the author, William A. Nelson, DC, a charter member of the ACA. The "so-called viral diseases," he stated, "follow the same general rule," with chiropractors deciding which children to refer to physicians. "We must not lose sight of the fact that . . . our therapy is preeminent in reestablishing normal physiology where such is possible."

According to Dr. Nelson, chiropractors can also evaluate heart problems in children. "If not an acute emergency," he advised, "the easiest way may well be a short period of trial treatment." The only conditions for which he stressed medical referral among children or adolescents were acute poisoning and venereal disease.

To CU's knowledge, there is only one United States or Canadian statute that recognizes any specific need to protect children under chiropractic treatment. That is a New York State law prohibiting chiropractors from X-raying anyone under age eighteen. The absence of any other safeguards represents, in CU's opinion, a tragic negligence on the part of legislators of both countries.

Chiropractors use X-rays to diagnose a disease process

that does not exist. Even if it did, though, X-rays would hardly help. Unlike bone, nerve tissue can't be seen on X-rays; nor do other fine details of soft tissues stand out. Hence, what chiropractors actually look for on X-rays are curvatures of the spine and departures from postural symmetry, however minor. Those are supposed to imply the presence of subluxations, which allegedly disturb nerve impulses.

But structural variations in a normal spine—and any movement or shift from a perfectly straight posture just before the X-ray—will also produce departures from symmetry. And those ordinary, inconsequential variations can look much the same as chiropractic "misalignments." Generally, the variations identified as misalignments by chiropractors are judged entirely normal by radiologists, who have much more extensive training in X-ray interpretation than chiropractors have. Thus, the chiropractor's X-ray diagnosis is twice removed from reality: It depends on unscientific appraisal of a nonexistent disease.

X-rays can, of course, show true bone abnormalities, such as a fracture or tumor. But the 14-by-36-inch film frequently used by chiropractors for examining posture does not produce good bone detail. So, unless the chiropractor takes a smaller and more detailed view as well, abnormalities that would preclude manipulation may be missed.

Many chiropractors agree that the large film gives too little detail and too much radiation exposure. Indeed, one chiropractor quoted in the March 1975 issue of *The ACA Journal of Chiropractic* contended that "the doctor who takes such films just does it to impress the patient."

Critics of chiropractic concur in that sentiment and often charge that chiropractic X-rays are a promotional gimmick rather than a diagnostic aid. Some chiropractic writings lend support to that allegation. A bald example appears in the 1947 edition of *Modern X-Ray Practice and Chiropractic Spinography*, by P. A. Remier, who in the mid-1960s was head of the X-ray department at Palmer College of Chiropractic. According to Remier, some of the reasons why chiropractors should X-ray "every case" were: "It promotes confidence. It creates interest among patients. It procures business. It attracts a better class of patients. It adds prestige in your community. It builds a reliable reputation."

Today, such an attitude toward radiation no longer prevails at Palmer College nor at the other two chiropractic schools CU visited. In general, the X-ray departments of those colleges appeared to teach and encourage techniques for reducing radiation exposure. But such improvements fail to get to the heart of the problem. The fact is that chiropractic X-rays for detecting "subluxations" do not serve a scientifically valid purpose. In CU's opinion *all* such radiation is unwarranted.

Although current figures are not available, a 1971 survey by *The Journal of Clinical Chiropractic* indicates that more than ten million X-rays were being taken by United States and Canadian chiropractors annually. About two million of those were the 14-by-36-inch type, which irradiates the body from the skull to the thigh, including the lens of the eye, the thyroid gland, bone marrow, and the reproductive organs—four areas considered among the most susceptible to radiation damage. Evidence shows that exposure to large amounts of X-ray increases the likelihood of cataracts, thyroid cancer, leukemia, and reproductive-cell damage. Public-health officials are particularly concerned about the radiation dose to reproductive organs, since damage to the genetic material is a potential source of harm to future generations.

"On the average, 3 percent of people in a medical practice

are X-rayed," says the Montreal children's hospitals' report. "For the chiropractor, the figure is over 90 percent." In addition, 14-by-36 full-trunk X-rays account for less than one in every ten thousand hospital X-rays, and the great majority of hospitals do not take full-trunk X-rays at all. In contrast, about one in five chiropractic X-rays is of this type.

According to a report prepared for the Canadian Association of Radiologists in May 1974, chiropractic use of full-trunk X-rays is the greatest source of unnecessary gonadal radiation in Canada (especially for women, whose reproductive organs cannot be shielded from the primary X-ray beam). And chiropractic X-rays were judged second only to medical and dental X-rays as the leading sources of manmade radiation exposure in North America today. In CU's view, that is an extremely high risk to take for placebo medicine.

Despite the dangers of unscientific treatment, chiropractors today enjoy wider leeway in their scope of practice than any other health practitioner except the physician. By comparison, other independent health-care providers must practice within far stricter limits. A dentist doesn't treat stomach ulcers. A psychologist doesn't order medication for a heart condition. An optometrist doesn't treat epilepsy. But chiropractors may often do all three. And they are permitted to offer treatment in specialties ranging from pediatrics to psychiatry—without having scientific training in any of them. Chiropractors have won that freedom without engaging in research or demonstrating professional capability in those fields. They have won it by one method alone: political action.

For years, grass-roots politics has been the lifeblood of chiropractic. By marshaling the support of chiropractic patients, the profession has often achieved an effective political voice in legislation affecting its licensure and services. And that voice has been its protection against science. Opponents of chiropractic come to legislative hearings with information, with scientific studies, and with the official endorsements of national organizations. Chiropractors come armed with votes.

The inclusion of chiropractic services under Medicare, after a seven-year campaign by chiropractors and their supporters, provides a classic example. Against the combined opposition of the AMA, the United States Department of Health, Education, and Welfare, the National Council of Senior Citizens, and numerous other groups, the chiropractic lobby emphasized one primary weapon: the mailbox. Congressional aides were reportedly astonished over the sacks of prochiropractic mail, which never seemed to diminish. It got the message across.

In its eighty year war with science, chiropractic has won the major battles. Its next goal is the inclusion of chiropractic under a national health-insurance program. In the past, the public's freedom to choose among health practitioners has been honored in legislation affecting chiropractors. CU believes that principle will be sustained if a national health-insurance bill emerges. Before such services are included, however, we think that public safety demands a searching review and thorough reform of chiropractic practices by appropriate state and federal agencies.

Recommendations

Overall, CU believes that chiropractic is a significant hazard to many patients. Current licensing laws, in our opinion, lend an aura of legitimacy to unscientific practices and serve to protect the chiropractor rather than the public. In effect, those laws allow persons with limited qualifications to practice medicine under another name.

We believe the public health would be better served if state and federal governments used their licensing powers and their power of the purse to restrict the chiropractor's scope of practice more effectively. Specifically, we think that licensing laws and federal health-insurance programs should limit chiropractic treatment to appropriate musculoskeletal complaints and ban *all* chiropractic use of X-rays and drugs, including nutritional supplements, for the purported treatment of disease. Above all, we would urge that chiropractors be prohibited from treating children; children do not have the freedom to reject unscientific therapy that their parents may mistakenly turn to in a crisis.

If you've been considering a chiropractor for the first time, we think you'd be safer to reconsider. Even if you are dissatisfied with your physician's treatment of a back problem, you can ask for a consultation with another physician, such as an orthopedist or physiatrist (a specialist in physical medicine). Then, if manipulative treatment were indicated, it could be performed by that specialist or by a physical therapist.

Despite this recommendation, we recognize that some persons will decide to use the services of a chiropractor. For those who do, and who wish to avoid some of the dubious practices that occur, we think some advice given to CU by chiropractic officials themselves may be helpful.

■ Avoid any practitioner who makes claims about cures, either orally or in advertising. Anyone who implies or promises guaranteed results from treatment should be held suspect.

■ Beware of chiropractors who ask you to sign a contract for services. A written agreement is not customary practice.

■ Reject anyone advertising free X-rays. Radiation should not be used as a lure.

- Ask whether the chiropractor refers patients to other health professions. If the answer is 'No'—or if the chiropractor disparages other professions or accepted treatment —walk out.
- Don't make advance payments. Most chiropractors have a flat office fee and don't offer "discounts" for prepayment. Nor is it accepted practice to charge extra for "units of treatment," such as manipulation, heat therapy, and the like. That should be included in the office fee.
- Don't be pressured by scare tactics, such as threats of "irreversible damage" if treatment isn't begun promptly. And watch out for those who encourage "intensive treatment" because "anything less would be a patch-up job." The intensive treatment may apply to your bank account.

CU would add one more precaution: See a physician as well and find out what he or she has to say about the problem.

How to Pay Less for Prescription Drugs

At Congressional hearings in March 1974, Senator Gaylord Nelson of Wisconsin told of the problems faced by one manufacturer of generic drugs—those marketed without a brand name. According to Senator Nelson, that manufacturer supplied a particular drug to a well-known company that resold it under a brand name. The manufacturer sold the identical drug by generic name directly to pharmacists at a small fraction of the price charged by the brand-name company. But the manufacturer had difficulty convincing physicians to prescribe the unbranded version. He told them that the two drugs had been made by the same process, at the same plant, on the same day; he showed them photographs of the two products as evidence. But to little avail. Doctors still preferred to prescribe the higher-priced brand-name version. The manufacturer considered inventing a brand name to slap on the label of his generic drug and boosting its price to the level of the more expensive version.

It may sound strange for a manufacturer to consider raising a price—rather than lowering it—as a way to stimulate sales. But in the topsy-turvy world of prescription-drug economics, it's not strange at all. A recent study of the price structure of the antibiotic market (see below) suggests that the manufacturer would be heading in a very profitable direction indeed.

One of every five prescriptions written in this country is for an antibiotic. Many antibiotics have been on the market long enough so that patents have expired and the products no longer enjoy the monopoly advantage that patents give to new drugs (see page 278). Widely used antibiotics can be divided into a relative handful of chemical types, many of which are sold both as brand-name drugs and as generics. Thus, if conditions for true price competition were ripe anywhere in the prescription-drug market, they would be ripe in the market for antibiotics. To determine how competition is working in the antibiotics business, Consumers Union helped finance a research study undertaken on this topic by the Council on Economic Priorities (CEP).

The CEP is a New York-based nonprofit organization that conducts research on the performance of corporations in such areas as environmental quality and consumer practices. Its antibiotic study,* published in January 1975, focused on the seven largest-selling antibiotics available from more than one manufacturer. These are penicillin VK, penicillin G, tetracycline, oxytetracycline, ampicillin, erythromycin, and chloramphenicol. To conduct its analysis, the CEP reviewed two important sets of figures com-

*"Resistant Prices: A Study of Competitive Strains in the Antibiotic Markets." A condensation of the study is available for $1 from Council on Economic Priorities, 84 Fifth Avenue, New York, N.Y. 10011.

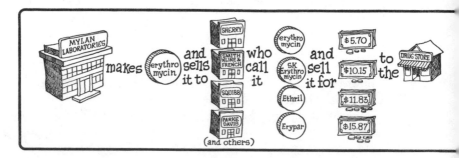

piled by IMS America, a market research firm. The first was each product's "average transaction price"—the average price at which the manufacturer sells the product to the pharmacist. (The price the consumer pays the pharmacist for a drug is on average about double the transaction price.) The second important statistic is the sales volume of each product.

The study's major finding: The brands of antibiotics that cost the most dominate the market. More prescriptions are written for them than for similar or identical (but less expensive) competitors, and thus they have greater volume of sales, both in terms of units and of dollars.

Consider the case of penicillin VK. According to the study, one of the most expensive brands of penicillin VK was Eli Lilly & Co.'s *V-cillin K;* it cost pharmacists $8.32 for 100 250-mg tablets—its most common dosage form and package size. *V-cillin K* (in all its sizes and forms) had drugstore sales of more than $22 million, or 54 percent of all sales of the drug. But druggists could also purchase 100 250-mg tablets of penicillin VK from Sherry Pharmaceutical Co. for just $1.85. The sales of Sherry's penicillin VK— the least expensive one available—were under $300,000 and thus too insignificant to be listed by IMS America.

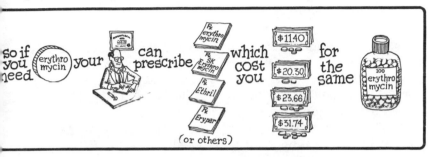

so if you need erythromycin your can prescribe Rx erythromycin, Rx SK Erythromycin, Rx Ethril, Rx Erypar (or others) which cost you $11.40 $20.30 $23.66 $31.74 for the same erythromycin

Sales of tetracycline presented another case in point. The study found that Lederle Laboratories' *Achromycin V*, one of the most expensive tetracyclines, controlled 29 percent of the market. More prescriptions were written for it than for any other tetracycline. The cheapest tetracycline, sold by H. L. Moore Drug Exchange Inc. for less than one-quarter the price of *Achromycin V*, had insignificant sales.

The story was similar for ampicillin and erythromycin. The most expensive ampicillin, *Polycillin*, sold by Bristol Laboratories, controlled the largest share of the market, 24 percent. Pfizer Laboratories' ampicillin, called *Pen A*, was less than half the price of *Polycillin* and had only 8 percent of the market.

Abbott Laboratories' *Erythrocin*, the highest-priced erythromycin product, controlled 60 percent of the market. Sherry's erythromycin, marketed to pharmacists for less than half *Erythrocin's* price, did not have significant sales.

If the above statistics indicate a problem with price competition in the market for those four antibiotics, consider the situation among the three remaining antibiotics: Squibb's *Pentids*, the most expensive penicillin G, had 78 percent of the sales of penicillin G. Pfizer's *Terramycin*, the most expensive oxytetracycline, had 99 percent of the sales of oxytetracycline. Parke, Davis & Co.'s *Chloromycetin,* the most expensive chloramphenicol, had 99 percent of the sales of chloramphenicol.*

Evidently, certain pharmaceutical firms have the market power to charge a price higher than their competition and still maintain sales. The CEP labeled that difference in price a "premium" that is granted to the larger firms. The premium is the difference between the lowest price at which the pharmacist can obtain the drug and the price charged by other suppliers of the same drug.

If Sherry sold penicillin VK for $1.85, for example, that price must at least have covered basic costs of manufacturing and distributing, or Sherry would have sold the product at a loss. It probably also included some money for profit. The extra $6.47 that Lilly charged for penicillin VK is a premium, presumably covering research activities, promotion, and other expenses, plus added profit. That $6.47 premium accounted for 78 percent of the total Lilly price of $8.32.

All told, the CEP estimated, at least 52 percent of the $173 million spent by pharmacies for the seven antibiotics was premium payment. That figures to more than $90 million in premium. Apparently, most prescription dollars are not going for the medication *in* the bottle but for the name *on it.*

In CU's view, most premium dollars are wasted dollars. They contribute neither to the quality of prescription drugs nor to the health of drug consumers.

The large, high-premium pharmaceutical firms argue

*There are clinical as well as competitive problems with chloramphenicol. Fatal cases of bone-marrow failure have been reported with use of that drug. Most medical authorities agree that chloramphenicol should be reserved for life-threatening infections. For a fuller report on the drug, see "The Peculiar Success of Chloromycetin," CONSUMER REPORTS, October 1970.

that their products are therapeutically superior to the products of other firms and are therefore worth a premium. Presumably, a firm selling under a brand name manufactures under its own controlled conditions and stands behind its own product. But things don't work that way in the real world of antibiotics, the CEP learned when it examined who manufactures what for whom. It found that Mylan Laboratories manufactured erythromycin in its final form for several firms, including Sherry, Smith Kline & French, Squibb, and Parke, Davis. Sherry's wholesale price for 100 250-mg tablets was $5.70; Smith Kline & French's was $10.15; Squibb's was $11.83; and Parke, Davis's $15.87. One manufacturer; four distributors, four different prices.

The ampicillin marketplace was stranger still. One company, Zenith Laboratories, Inc., manufactured the final dosage form for six other companies, which then charged from $4.40 to $8.60 for 100 250-mg capsules of the drug. Another manufacturer, Bristol Laboratories, put up ampicillin for three firms, with a price variation from $7.50 to $14.80. Oddly enough, the lowest price charged for the Bristol product, $7.50, and the highest price, $14.80, were both charged by the same firm, ICN Pharmaceuticals. The lower price was charged by its generic division and the higher price by its brand-name division. The same company can thus buy its product from the same source its competitors do and then proceed to sell the product for less than its competitors' price—and for more.

Dr. Henry Simmons, former director of the Food and Drug Administration's Bureau of Drugs, offered further evidence that brand names do not signify better drugs. All antibiotics are batch-certified by the Food and Drug Administration (FDA) for potency, purity, and stability. "Based on many years of experience with this program," said Dr. Simmons, "we are confident that there is no significant difference between so-called generic and brand-name antibiotic products on the American market." On the basis of FDA studies of nineteen other classes of drugs, "we cannot conclude there is a significant difference in quality between the generic and brand-name product tested." Dr. Simmons pointed out that defects have been encountered in both brand and generic products manufactured by large and small companies.

The CEP examined recall data for antibiotics from January 1971 through July 1974. Those recalls indicate that major firms do not have a better record than small firms.

There is another question that bears on therapeutic superiority. The Pharmaceutical Manufacturers Association (PMA), an organization whose 110 member companies are responsible for approximately 95 percent of all prescription-drug sales in this country, claims that products that are chemically equivalent (that contain the same amounts of the same active ingredients in the same dosage form) may not be *therapeutically* equivalent. That is, they may not be equally effective in treating the patient's disease.

An important factor in determining therapeutic equivalence is bioavailability—the amount of the product's active ingredient that is absorbed into the bloodstream to perform its function. Bioavailability may be affected by many factors, including particle size and shape, and the nature of the so-called inert ingredients contained in the drug product. If two drugs have the same bioavailability, they are termed *bioequivalent*.

The scientific issue of bioavailability has generated a controversy in the drug industry because of its economic implications. If chemically equivalent drugs are also therapeutically equivalent, there would seem to be no reason for physicians to prescribe a brand-name drug with a "premium" price rather than a cheaper generic version.

The controversy became a significant public issue in December 1973, when Caspar Weinberger, then Secretary of the Department of Health, Education, and Welfare (HEW), said his department planned to limit reimbursement for any drug under Medicare and Medicaid "to the lowest cost at which the drug is generally available unless there is a demonstrated difference in therapeutic effect." The reaction of the PMA was quick and critical. Its president, C. Joseph Stetler, termed the proposal a "huge gamble" that could endanger the health of the elderly and the poor. Beneficiaries of Medicaid and Medicare, he said, would be forced to accept drugs that were not therapeutically equivalent to established brand-name drugs.

To settle the issue, a report on drug bioequivalence was prepared by a panel organized by the Office of Technology Assessment (OTA), a Congressional investigative body. The panel, chaired by Dr. Robert Berliner, Dean of the Yale University School of Medicine, reported in July 1974 that variations in bioavailability *have* been demonstrated in chemically equivalent products in a number of drug categories. Those variations have been responsible for a few documented therapeutic failures. Most notably, several different brands of digoxin (a highly potent drug used for treating cardiac failure and certain abnormal cardiac rhythms) were found to differ in bioavailability. Levels of digoxin in the blood just twice as high as therapeutic levels can cause serious, even fatal, reactions. Too little digoxin can also be dangerous, as the dose is then inadequate for therapy. Digoxin is now undergoing batch-by-batch certification by the FDA, and every company marketing the drug must present evidence of bioavailability.

Differences in bioavailability, although not necessarily therapeutic inequivalence, have been documented for a number of other drugs, including diphenylhydantoin, an anticonvulsant; phenylbutazone, an anti-inflammatory drug; prednisone, a cortisone analogue; and tolbutamide, an oral hypoglycemic agent.

But for most drugs, the gap between therapeutic dose and toxic dose is wider than for digoxin, and any differences in bioavailability would not be so critical. The OTA panel concluded that the great proportion of chemically equivalent products—85 to 90 percent, according to Dr. Berliner's estimate—presents no problems of therapeutic equivalency and could be used interchangeably. "Most drugs ought to be prescribed generically," Dr. Berliner told CU.

With the controversy over bioequivalence at last put in perspective, HEW went ahead with its plans for lowest-cost reimbursement, which took effect in August 1976. The program provides for a pharmaceutical reimbursement board to set a maximum allowable cost (MAC) that the federal government will pay for prescription drugs available from more than one supplier. Cost limits would be imposed only on drug products that do not present problems of therapeutic equivalency. The FDA expects to have ready before the end of 1976 regulations for identifying and listing inequivalent drugs and for requiring bioavailability data for any drug that is potentially inequivalent.

Meanwhile, HEW has proceeded to implement MAC. In September 1976, HEW initiated the process by which the pharmaceutical reimbursement board would establish the cost limit for a drug under MAC. Ampicillin was the first drug chosen (antibiotics being already certified for bioequivalence). The flow of MAC prices that HEW anticipates will follow in ampicillin's wake may be impeded by legal action, still unresolved as of this writing. (In 1975, the American Medical Association—later joined by the PMA—filed suit in Federal District Court in Chicago to block the MAC program.)

Also part of the lowest-cost reimbursement program is EAC (estimated acquisition cost), which provides that drug-reimbursing agencies—primarily the states under Medicaid—establish an EAC for prescription drugs as well as specify the dispensing fee a pharmacist may charge to fill the prescription. If the MAC price for a multi-source drug should be lower than the EAC rate, however, MAC would prevail since the regulations require that only the lowest cost be reimbursed. To facilitate EAC, HEW compiles and distributes to the states a comparative survey of drug prices.

In addition to bioequivalence, the high-premium firms have offered another justification for their premiums: The extra price helps cover the cost of the scientific work that goes into the development of new drugs. Basic scientific work is risky business, they contend, and high risk justifies high profits.

The profits have indeed been high. Over the past decade the drug industry has ranked as one of the two most profitable manufacturing industries in the country (the other is soft drinks). In 1973, the profit rate on stockholders' equity after taxes was 18.9 percent for drug manufacturers, compared with 12.8 percent for all manufacturing corporations. And the pharmaceutical industry had a 9.4 percent return on sales, the second highest (after mining) and more than double the average for all industries.

What about the risk? According to an HEW task force that reported on prescription drugs in 1968, "The exceptionally high rate of profit which generally marks the drug industry is not accompanied by any peculiar degree of risk or by any unique difficulties in obtaining growth capital." The top firms have been remarkably stable, and their earnings have grown steadily—signs that the industry is relatively risk-free.

It is true that the prescription-drug industry spends heavily for research. According to the PMA, the drug industry spends five times as much of its sales income for research as does American industry as a whole. And the bulk of the research is done by large firms that sell brand-name drugs.

The HEW task force was not overly impressed by the quality of that research. The task force characterized it as a "waste of skilled research manpower and research facilities," a "waste of chemical facilities needed to test the products," and responsible for a "confusing proliferation of drug products which are promoted to physicians"—all of which results in a "further burden on the taxpayer who in the long run must pay the cost." In an FDA study of more than eight hundred drugs introduced in the United States between 1950 and 1973, two-thirds were found to represent little or no therapeutic gain over existing drugs.

The PMA estimated the cost of basic research (creating new chemical entities) at $100 million in 1971 and the cost of research and development as a whole (including modifying already existing drugs and testing drugs to meet FDA requirements) at $629 million. Those outlays sound high, but they don't measure up to the more than $1 billion the industry spends each year on promotion—persuading physicians that brand A is better than brand B, and that generic nonbrand X just doesn't do the job.

Companies that carry on research and develop new drugs should be rewarded for their contributions to medical progress and human welfare. And they are—by the patent system. The company that has developed a new drug enjoys for seventeen years exclusive rights to produce and sell it and to license production and sales to other firms for a fee. (According to the PMA, the life of a patent is actually only ten and a half years because of regulatory requirements that delay marketing after the patent has been granted. It has been estimated, however, that most patent drugs pay off the cost of research and development in their first three years on the market.)

Prices and premiums are generally highest during the time of patent-protected monopoly. But even after the patent expires, the original drug usually enjoys such a great advantage that effective price competition is stymied.

That advantage is rooted in the brand-name system. While a drug is undergoing clinical investigation, it is given its *generic* name by the United States Adopted Names Council (a semiofficial organization sponsored by the American Medical Association, the United States Pharmacopeial Convention, and the American Pharmaceutical Association). When the drug is ready for marketing, it is given its *brand* name by the pharmaceutical firm and that name is registered as a trademark. In many cases, generic names are chemical tongue-twisters whereas brand names are short, simple, and catchy—designed to be remembered easily by physicians.

A patent-holder retains the right to the original brand name after the patent expires. Competing companies must invent their own brand names or market the drug under its generic name. But a drug by any other name doesn't sell the same. The patent-holder typically uses the patent period, and the revenues derived from monopoly pricing, to mount a massive promotional campaign aimed not only at selling the drug under its brand name while the patent lasts but also at linking that name with the product permanently, so that physicians will continue to prescribe the drug by its original brand name long after the patent period has elapsed. Thus it is that doctors who want to prescribe a sleeping pill may well think first of *Nembutal*, the brand name that Abbott Laboratories pushed without competition for the length of its patent. The generic name, pentobarbital, may not even come to mind. Yet many smaller companies sell their versions of pentobarbital at a fraction of the price charged for *Nembutal*.

To try to catch up to the early favorite, manufacturers of equivalent brand-name products also spend large sums on promotion. Like the manufacturer holding the patent, they give presents to medical students and doctors; they sponsor medical conferences; they advertise in medical journals and magazines; they publish quasi-medical literature in the form of newspapers and circulars.

At Senate hearings, twenty leading manufacturers said they distributed more than 2 billion free drug samples to physicians and other professionals in 1973. They also said they distributed some 13 million gifts valued at more than $5 million and 45 million "reminders," such as calendars and rulers, valued at more than $8 million. More than three thousand plant tours were conducted at a cost exceeding $748,000. According to testimony by former industry "detail men"—sort of door-to-door salespersons who promote drug products directly to physicians and pharmacists—freezers, color television sets, bicycles, and camping equipment were offered to doctors and druggists in return for prescribing or buying particular brand-name products.

The drug industry spends an average of $5,000 per private practitioner to promote brand-name prescribing. As one result, although about 35 percent of drugs are no longer under patent, only some 10 percent of prescriptions are written generically rather than for a specific brand name. And yet brand-name drugs often cost five to ten times more than their generic counterparts—and sometimes up to thirty times more. According to T. Donald Rucker, former head of the Social Security Administration's drug studies unit, the high degree of product loyalty created by promotion directly to physicians is "a dominant factor enabling pharmaceutical manufacturers to exercise control over drug prices."

That control is extended by antisubstitution laws. In many states, pharmacists must fill a prescription with the exact brand ordered by the physician, even though they may also stock a cheaper, equivalent version of the same drug. If a prescription is written generically, a pharmacist may fill it with either a brand-name or generic version of the drug. Some pharmacists apply a fixed service fee to the basic cost of the drug product. Others charge for their services by adding a fixed percentage to the cost of the prescription. The fixed-percentage markup encourages pharmacists to dispense a high-priced brand-name drug even when a doctor prescribes by generic name. Also, pharmacists can keep their inventory costs down by stocking only one or two of the largest-selling brand names and using them to fill both brand-name and generic prescriptions.

At each stage of the process that brings drugs from the scientist's laboratory to patients, there now exists restraints that limit price competition, keeping drug prices higher than they should be. The patent system provides protection for a new drug for seventeen years; the brand-name system, bolstered by promotional blitzes and antisubstitution requirements, protects established, brand-name drugs after the patent period elapses. And retail practices may thwart any savings the doctor may make possible by prescribing generically.

The antisubstitution barrier, however, has now been breached. After a two-year study, the Drug Research Board of the National Research Council recommended in January 1975 that pharmacists be allowed to substitute for a brand-name drug a less-expensive generic equivalent unless a physician specifically indicates no substitution is to be made.

According to the Drug Research Board, "The pharmacist may, in some situations, have greater knowledge of drug products than other health professionals, including knowledge of both quality and costs."

Twenty states and the District of Columbia now permit some form of drug substitution. Provisions of these generic substitution laws vary widely, however. Some are so restrictive that substitution-minded pharmacists could be handcuffed by a state's purportedly pro-substitution regulations. For example, a proviso that substitutions must be limited to drugs certified by the FDA as bioequivalent effectively protects all brand-name prescription drugs except antibiotics.

In July 1976, the Federal Trade Commission (FTC) authorized an investigation of drug substitution laws to uncover any unfair or deceptive practices in sales to consumers of multi-source drugs. According to the staff attorney in charge of the investigation, the FTC hopes to study how drug substitution actually works in the twenty states permitting the practice and whether consumers benefit in dollar savings. The impact of antisubstitution laws in the remaining states will also be assessed. At the conclusion of its investigation, which could take until the end of 1977, the FTC may recommend that a trade regulation be enacted facilitating generic substitution.

Over the past few years, legislation has been introduced in Congress designed to compensate for business practices that keep the prices of prescription drugs unrealistically high. There have been bills in both houses, for example, that would modify the patent system. Manufacturers of new drugs would be required to license other companies to make those drugs if exorbitant pricing practices occurred during the patent period. Legislation has been introduced in the Senate to ban drug-company gifts to physicians and pharmacists; establish a national drug testing and evaluation center; and require the federal government to publish a National Drug Compendium containing therapeutic and price information. The FDA has already begun work on a drug compendium, scheduled for publication sometime after 1978. The FDA does not plan, however, to include price information—a serious omission, in CU's view.

Bills were introduced in the House to repeal all state antisubstitution laws and in the Senate to require prescription-drug labels to bear the manufacturer's name and address, so the person who takes the drug will know whether the brand-name distributor was also the actual manufacturer of the product.

Those measures all strike at features of the prescription-drug industry that are conducive to overpricing, and they all deserve consumer support. But the best legislative medicine for consumers is a bill that Senator Gaylord Nelson plans to reintroduce in the new Congress. It would eliminate brand names from prescription drugs. Under its provisions, a drug would be prescribed and sold under its generic name only, although a physician could still specify a particular *manufacturer* on a prescription. When no maker is singled out, the use of generic names should help the consumer purchase the least expensive equivalent drug the pharmacist has. (Since 1974 the American Pharmaceutical Association has supported the elimination of brand names for all prescription drugs.)

Such a law would help loosen the stranglehold that large, brand-name manufacturers have over the prescription-drug market. First of all, it would take the steam (and the expense) out of their promotional efforts. Why push a drug if a score of other companies are making the same drug and if there's no brand name to distinguish yours from theirs? And it would take the steam out of the antisubstitution laws that so often prevent consumers from obtaining cheaper, equivalent therapy.

The main goal of drug therapy, of course, is not lower prices but better health. Senator Nelson's bill would contribute to that goal by eliminating a source of therapeutic confusion. For every prescription drug there is an average of thirty names—aliases that can obscure the identity of the medication not only from patients but from prescribing physicians.

Canada, though far behind the United States in developing new drugs, is well ahead in developing ways to reduce drug prices. Canada passed a compulsory drug licensing law in 1969. Under it, a company can apply to the government for permission to produce a drug that is still under patent. And several Canadian provinces have passed "product selection" laws permitting pharmacists to substitute for a doctor's prescribed drug either a generic or brand-name equivalent.

In 1970, the province of Ontario implemented a unique, voluntary program called Parcost (Prescriptions at a Reasonable Cost). At its core is a Comparable Drug Index—listings of interchangeable drugs that have passed quality tests and are arranged in order of descending price. Drug quality is evaluated by a committee of medical and drug experts who inspect manufacturing plants and analyze drug samples. Where an equivalency problem is discovered, the Index indicates that the products involved are not interchangeable.

When an Ontario pharmacist substitutes for a prescribed brand-name drug, the substitute product must be one listed in the Index and must be lower in cost than the prescribed product. A generically written prescription must be filled with the lowest-priced interchangeable drug in a pharmacist's inventory.

All Ontario druggists must abide by those substitution rules. More than half the pharmacists in Ontario have also agreed to charge the patient a fixed professional fee for dispensing rather than a percentage mark-up. (The maximum dispensing fee is now set at $2.75.)

If nothing else, the program appears to have made Ontario physicians conscious of the cost of medications. In 1973, the latest year for which data are available, about one-third of the prescriptions for drugs marketed by more than one drug company were written generically, up 6 percent from the year before. Another 31 percent were written for brands lower in cost than the most expensive, up 2 percent from 1972.

Recommendations

Until a rational drug marketplace is developed in the United States, consumers must fend for themselves when buying prescription drugs. To help you cut prescription costs now, CU offers the following advice.

Ask your doctor to prescribe a drug by its generic name. As we noted earlier, generic drugs tend to be substantially less expensive than brand-name drugs. Although a pharmacist may not actually sell you the least expensive form of the drug, the CEP study uncovered this interesting fact: Pharmacists often charge less for a generic prescription than for a brand-name prescription *even when the same product from the same manufacturer is used to fill both.*

Ask your doctor to specify the manufacturer who sells the cheapest equivalent product. That will ensure the lowest-cost therapy, provided the druggist passes on the savings. Unfortunately, price information has not been readily available to doctors. But they can try to obtain it by consulting pharmacists, pharmaceutical company representatives, and by obtaining catalogs from generic drug companies. Beginning in 1977, the price information collected to implement MAC/EAC will be distributed twice a year to all physicians and pharmacists and made available to the general public through the Government Printing Office.

If you are going to continue a specific drug for a long period, ask your doctor to prescribe it in a large quantity. Large-quantity prescriptions are generally more economical and will save repeated trips to the pharmacy. Be sure to check the expiration date of the product with the druggist. If the date will fall before you are scheduled to use up the drug, you should buy a smaller quantity. To preserve the life of a drug as long as possible, ask the pharmacist about the best method of storage.

Shop around. Numerous surveys, including CU's ("What's the Price of an Rx Drug?" CONSUMER REPORTS, May 1970), have documented a wide difference in drug prices from store to store in the same city. Your chances of getting price information may have been helped by a recent Supreme Court decision. Before May 1976, when a Virginia law prohibiting pharmacists from advertising prescription-drug prices was ruled unconstitutional, there were thirty-three states with similar limitations on advertising drug prices. But in some areas—until pharmacists use their new right to advertise—you may still have to shop for price. If you prefer to shop by telephone, you may be able to find out drug price information without leaving your home. Organizations that are interested in consumer issues may wish to conduct price surveys of commonly prescribed drugs at local pharmacies.

If it's not an emergency situation, ask a number of pharmacists the cost of a prescription before you have it filled. If it's a generic prescription without a manufacturer specified, ask for the least expensive version of the drug.

If you live in California, Connecticut, Maryland, Michigan, Minnesota, Nevada, New Hampshire, New York, Texas, Vermont, or the city of Boston, your drug shopping will be made somewhat easier by posters listing the prices of the top-selling prescription drugs (though you may have trouble ferreting out the posters in some stores). Mandatory price-posting is being enforced in those ten states and Boston; in Maine, South Dakota, West Virginia, and the District of Columbia, mandatory price-posting has been legislated and is in the process of implementation, as of this writing. In Hawaii and Washington, price-posting is permitted but not required. In any case, if your prescription is for a drug not listed on the poster, you will still have to ask for its price.

Wherever you live, inquire about discounts sometimes given routinely to the elderly and to other special categories of patients—but first find out the regular consumer price.

The FDA has acted to standardize drug information in those states where pharmacies post or advertise prescription drug prices. Since January 1976, pharmacies must specify the generic and brand name (if any) of a drug, its dosage strength and dosage form, and the price charged for a specific quantity. The quoted price must include all charges to the consumer, such as the cost of the drug, dispensing fees charged by the pharmacist, and handling charges (if any).

While this report has emphasized drug prices, you should also consider what pharmaceutical services you want—credit, home delivery, personal attention, twenty-four-hour availability in case of emergency, records of your purchases, for example. Such services may be available only at pharmacies that price prescriptions on the high side to cover the extra expense. Only you can decide if such services are worth higher prices.

How to Buy a Hearing Aid

WHAT CONSUMERS SHOULD KNOW

In 1970, after lengthy litigation, Consumers Union forced the Veterans Administration (VA) to reveal its ratings of hearing aids—ratings based on data developed at public expense and, therefore, under the 1967 Freedom of Information Act, open to public disclosure. It was, as we noted at the time, a narrow victory for consumers. For one thing, the government agency limited its application of the principle of disclosure to hearing aids. For another, the information that was revealed was of direct benefit only to hearing specialists, not to people in need of aids.

The next year, in 1971, when we published the VA ratings (as we do the most recent ratings at the end of this report), we commented on serious shortcomings in the system of manufacture, marketing, and fitting of hearing aids. The extent of the difficulties that plague the hard-of-hearing could only be guessed at in 1971. The focus is sharper now, thanks to a monumental report by the Department of Health, Education, and Welfare (HEW) Interdepartmental Task Force on Hearing Aids, reports by public-interest groups, and hearings before the United States Senate Subcommittee on Consumer Interests of the Elderly. The picture that has emerged from those reports and hearings is very discouraging indeed.

The HEW Task Force reported that 14.5 million persons in the United States suffer some form of hearing impairment, but more than 10 million of those have received no medical attention for their disability. Yet, paradoxically, a significant number of the approximately 600,000 Americans who do buy hearing aids each year either don't need the aids, receive no benefit from them, or would be better served by medical or surgical treatment.

It's a pity that the vast majority of persons with impaired hearing receive no professional help. As we noted back in 1971, even partial deafness causes enormous problems. Children with such a handicap are sometimes mistakenly marked down as slow-witted, and they may have behavioral problems. Adults may suffer strained relations with those forced to shout or repeat themselves. People of any age risk physical danger from things they can't hear.

It's not hard to understand why hearing loss so often goes uncorrected. Hard-of-hearing persons may try to conceal their condition for fear it will set them back professionally or socially. Vanity may play a role, too, in the form of an effort to deny any disability. Ignorance of the kind of help available is another factor. But, certainly, one important reason many people remain unhelped is the high—possibly unreasonably high—price of hearing aids.

In terms of technical complexity, a hearing aid isn't much different from the audio-amplifier section of an ordinary transistor radio, with a microphone added. But aids cost $350 and more. Why?

The HEW Task Force reported that the parts in a $350

hearing aid cost $30. The costs for labor, advertising, and promotion run about $45, bringing the total manufacturer's cost to $75. The manufacturer sells the aid to a dealer for between $80 and $140. The dealer then tags on a 200 to 300 percent markup. Those are huge markups, raising the question of why competitive forces have failed to hold them in check. The Federal Trade Commission (FTC) provided some answers after a full investigation of the hearing-aid industry.

Among the findings of FTC staff members: The four largest hearing-aid manufacturers account for 50 percent of all hearing-aid shipments; the eight largest, 70 percent. Such high market shares in any one industry indicate what economists refer to as a shared monopoly, or oligopoly. An oligopolized industry tends not to compete on price and quality, the product characteristics important to consumers. It tends to compete instead in promotion, especially promotion designed to "differentiate" one manufacturer's product from a competitor's essentially similar product.

In 1975, the FTC accused six hearing-aid makers of, among other things, falsely claiming that their devices were new inventions or that they embodied new engineering concepts. Even though all six of the manufacturers agreed by July 1976 to end such claims, there's little hope for lasting improvement. Similar FTC actions in the past against many of the same manufacturers failed to clean up such practices.

Turning to retail dealers, the FTC found competition as constricted there as among maufacturers. Manufacturers sell aids directly to dealers. Some dealers carry only a single brand of hearing aid and are granted exclusive selling territories by the manufacturer. The dealers handle only one brand, according to complaints by the FTC against five manufacturers, because the factories coerce and intimidate them into doing so. (Four of the manufacturers, Sonotone Corporation, Radioear Corporation, Dahlberg Electronics, Inc., and the Maico Hearing Instruments Division of Textron, Inc., signed consent orders with the FTC agreeing to stop the restrictive practices. Beltone Electronics Corporation has decided to appeal a September 1976 ruling by an FTC administrative law judge that the company's practices are in restraint of trade.)

With only one brand to sell, dealers are subject to great pressure from manufacturers, who may prove adamant about the maintenance of artificially constructed list prices. According to FTC complaints, hearing-aid manufacturers have threatened to stop supplying dealers who cut prices. But most dealers have little cause to abandon their high markups. An estimated 7,900 dealers sell a total of 600,000 hearing aids each year. Most dealers, therefore, sell very few each year, but those few go at high prices.

What to do about it? There are a few faint glimmerings of reform in the marketing and pricing of hearing aids, which we'll touch on later. But for now—and indeed at any time—it's best to remember that hearing loss is, above all, a medical problem. And, as in 1971, our best advice on seeking a remedy begins with a basic understanding of that fact.

Loss of hearing may be caused by a number of things: accumulation of earwax, infection in the ear, certain diseases (such as measles or meningitis), a reaction to antibiotics, tumors, a head injury, a birth defect, long exposure to high sound levels. Perhaps the most common cause of all is a condition called presbycusis, part of the aging process. Few persons over sixty-five can hear as well as they did when they were twenty-five.

Whatever the specific cause, there are two broad categories into which all hearing loss falls—"conductive" and "sensorineural." Conductive loss results from a failure in some part of the physical linkage of tissue and bones that conducts sound impulses from the eardrum to the nerve centers of the inner ear. A conductive hearing loss usually blocks and muffles sound uniformly, similar to when you cover your ear with your hand. Sensorineural loss results from damage to the nerve centers in the inner ear, the nerve pathways to the brain, or perhaps to that portion of the brain that receives and interprets audio nerve signals. It's characterized by the inability to hear particular sound frequencies or tones, which may lead to difficulty in understanding certain words and sounds used in normal speech. For example, "s" may be confused with "f" because the nerve fibers that differentiate them are affected. Sensorineural loss is also frequently accompanied by increased sensitivity to loud sounds, which gives discomfort or pain, and by humming and buzzing sensations. It's not at all uncommon for a person who is hard of hearing to be suffering from both kinds of loss.

Most conductive losses can be corrected by surgery. But very few sensorineural losses can be corrected surgically or medically. People with sensorineural loss usually have no other recourse than to be fitted with a hearing aid, which will be helpful in many, but not all, cases.

If you have difficulty hearing, the first thing to do is to consult a medical doctor—preferably your family physician —who may decide that the problem calls for a specialist. In that case you'll probably be referred to an otolaryngologist or otologist. An otolaryngologist is a physician specializing in ear, nose, and throat problems. An otologist is a physician who specializes in ear problems only. (In the interest of simplicity, we'll use the term otologist to describe both kinds of specialists.) It is possible, of course, to go directly to an otologist; you can find the names of those practicing nearest you by calling your local medical society. The important point is to seek competent medical help.

More can be at stake than the loss of hearing. Oncoming deafness is occasionally due to serious pathology close to the body's path of hearing—a tumor, for instance. A medical diagnosis, then, could be of lifesaving importance.

To determine whether a hearing aid may help you, a specialist will take a detailed medical history and perform a complete evaluation of your ears, nose, and throat. You may then undergo hearing tests in the specialist's office or be referred to an audiologist. Audiologists are nonmedical, university-trained specialists who are skilled in evaluative and rehabilitative services for people with hearing problems.

A reliable indicator of an audiologist's skills is a Certificate of Clinical Competence issued by the American Speech and Hearing Association (ASHA), the professional body that governs the field of audiology. That certificate should not be confused with the designation of Certified Hearing Aid Audiologist displayed by many hearing-aid dealers and granted by the National Hearing Aid Society, the dealers' trade association. A certified member of ASHA has had to comply with much sterner training requirements than a member of the trade association.

One hitch in the recommended course is that it may take time and effort to get professional help. While there is no longer an absolute shortage of otologists and certified clinical audiologists, few are located in rural areas. A second hitch is that professional help may cost a sizable sum. Fees vary throughout the country, of course. In the Washington, D.C., area, an otologist's examination could cost $25. A hearing test and hearing-aid evaluation done at a hospital-connected speech and hearing clinic would cost another $45 to $60, making a total of $70 to $85. An otologist in a Los

Angeles suburb told us he charges $22 for an initial medical checkup and $10 for a hearing test on the second visit. The audiologist with whom he works then charges $45 for a hearing-aid evaluation. Although these examples may not be typical for all areas, they indicate that it's not unusual to pay $80 or more for a proper introduction to a hearing aid.

In certain areas, though, the introductory professional fees need not be extra expenses. A number of otologists and audiologists refer patients who need hearing aids to dealers who (despite the displeasure of manufacturers) have agreed to provide discounts. The dealers do so because they're spared the expense of evaluation and testing. The director of one hearing clinic in Washington, D.C., told CU that, because of such discounts, his patients pay no more for professional services and an aid than they would for an aid alone from most local dealers. The Los Angeles otologist told us that he arranges a 10 percent discount with a local dealer. That often covers the $45 charged by his associated audiologist for a hearing-aid evaluation.

The battery of tests in an audiological examination are generally of two types. One type employs an electrical device called an audiometer to determine the patient's ability to detect pure tones of various pitches. The second type investigates the patient's comprehension of certain spoken words.

Both the pure-tone and spoken-word tests are performed with varying degrees of sound intensity, usually measured in decibels (dB). The number of decibels of a sound is derived logarithmically from the number of times that sound is stronger than the weakest sound audible to the normal ear. The more decibels, the stronger the sound.

Among other things, the ear specialist tests for two important limits at frequencies deemed important for speech intelligibility: the threshold of hearing and the threshold of discomfort. Your threshold of hearing is the weakest sound that you can hear. Your threshold of discomfort is the loudest sound that you can hear without distress. A sound slightly louder than your threshold of discomfort marks your threshold of pain, the point at which your ear will hurt. A person with normal hearing has a threshold of hearing near 0 dB and a threshold of discomfort of about 120 dB. In tests for loss of hearing, an elevation of the threshold of hearing is generally the most significant finding. The table below shows how, as the threshold shifts upward in the general speech frequency range, the degree of impairment becomes more severe.

Threshold Shift (dB)	Characterization	Effect
0-15 (in the poorer ear)	Normal	No difficulties
15-30 (in the better ear)	Near normal	Difficulty with faint speech
30-45 (in the better ear)	Mild impairment	Difficulty with normal speech
45-60 (in the better ear)	Moderate impairment	Difficulty with loud speech
60-90 (in the better ear)	Severe impairment	Can understand only amplified speech
90 or more (in the better ear)	Profound impairment	Difficulty even with amplified speech

With some conductive losses, the range from the threshold of hearing to the threshold of discomfort decreases by the same number of decibels in all frequencies. With others, the threshold of discomfort shifts upward, so that one can tolerate louder sounds than previously.

Sensorineural hearing losses can be more complicated. Often, the threshold of hearing shifts differently for different frequencies. Thus, you might be able to hear a bass tone normally, a mid-range tone starting at 30 dB, and a high treble starting at 50 dB. To further complicate matters, the threshold of discomfort is apt to fall. Persons so afflicted may ask you to speak louder because they can't hear you; then, when you raise your voice moderately, it seems to them you're shouting. There are still other variations in sensorineural loss—for example, "holes" or gaps in the audible frequency range that prevent certain isolated tones from being heard normally. Complex and patternless sensorineural losses make the specification of an aid extremely difficult.

Adding to the difficulty are as yet unresolved questions in hearing-aid technology: Should an aid be designed to give the wearer tonally even sound, by strongly amplifying only those tones heard most poorly? Or will an aid work just as well if it provides equal amplification of all frequencies, or perhaps a moderate emphasis in the treble tones? Hearing specialists do not agree on the answers to those questions.

The important components of a hearing aid are a microphone to pick up the sound, an amplifier to boost the loudness of the sound, a receiver (or earphone) to deliver the sound, and a battery as a power source. Nearly all aids in use are air-conduction types, which put the sound directly into the ear canal through a molded ear piece. Bone-conduction aids, which direct the sound against the skull (usually the mastoid bone behind the ear), have limited application.

Four styles of air-conduction aids are in common use. The smallest is worn *in* the ear. Because it's so tiny, it can't provide powerful amplification; it's for cases of mild or moderate hearing loss. The largest and most powerful aids are worn on the body, in a front pocket or pinned to a garment, with only the receiver extending by wire to the ear.

However, body aids can pick up rustling noise from the user's clothing, or sound may be blocked by heavy over-clothing.

But 80 percent of the hearing aids in use are of moderate size and intermediate power. They fall into two types: behind-the-ear (or over-the-ear) aids, the familiar half-moon shaped apparatus worn between the ear and head; and eyeglass aids, contained in the temple of the eyeglass frame.

The useful amplification of a hearing aid is referred to as "average gain," measured in decibels over normal voice frequencies. A conventional aid with an average gain of 50 dB, which would put it in the moderate-power class, can amplify sound 50 dB. Conventional aids are classified in three power categories: strong (as high as 65 dB), moderate, and mild (as low as 29 dB).

To prevent pain and damage to the ear, aids have a limit to the loudness they can produce. That limit is called the "saturation sound-pressure level" or "maximum power output," also measured in decibels. It's usually set around the threshold of discomfort. Thus, if an aid with an average gain of 60 dB and a maximum power output of 120 dB receives a sound of 80 dB, it won't boost that sound to 140 dB, but rather cut it off at 120 dB. The average gain and maximum power output needed by any one person is determined in the audiological evaluation, although even those averages will not fully describe a hearing loss that is different for different frequencies.

There are specialty models with features designed to compensate for particular kinds of hearing loss:

With *compression models*, the gain isn't equal at all levels. Strong sounds are amplified less than weak sounds.

Directional models do not amplify sounds from the rear as much as they do from the front, helping the wearer to discriminate between desirable sounds and background noise.

High-frequency-emphasis models emphasize the treble, providing little or no amplification below 100 Hertz (Hz), or cycles per second.

The *CROS model* differs from conventional aids in that its microphone is placed on the opposite side of the head from the receiver. Originally designed for people with a hearing loss in only one ear, it has proved of benefit to people with bilateral losses, too. One of its major advantages is that when it's used with an earpiece with an opening there is a marked reduction of low-frequency background noise.

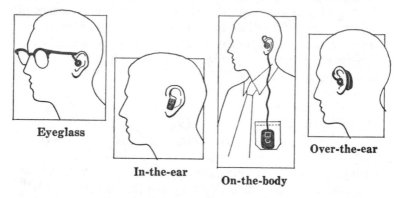

Eyeglass

In-the-ear

On-the-body

Over-the-ear

With *BICROS* models a microphone is placed on each side of the head, and signals from both microphones are delivered to one ear. Such models are of benefit to persons with unequal amounts of hearing loss in each ear.

Even when an aid is well fitted and working properly, most first-time users go through a period of adjustment because sounds are different when heard with the use of a hearing aid. The quality of sound, especially nonspeech sound, is more "brassy" than normal, in part because of the hearing aid's limited frequency range. It takes close to the full range of normal hearing, about 50 Hz to 10,000 Hz, to provide reasonably accurate timbre (the quality given to sound by its overtones), whereas most hearing aids work in a narrower range of about 500 to 4,000 Hz, which is sufficient to make sound intelligible but not entirely natural. Sounds are further distorted because hearing aids don't handle all tones evenly. And many people with hearing aids find themselves unable to "tune out" distracting sounds, as a person with normal hearing does—everything from a slamming door to a jet flying overhead seems unnaturally loud and jarring. With patience, however, and perhaps rehabilitative therapy with a qualified audiologist, most people can adjust to the imperfections of hearing aids.

Even those who seek to remedy their hearing loss in the recommended, medically directed way have no guarantee of success. In a sense, they start with four strikes against them.

First, the degree and quality of hearing loss can be difficult to determine precisely, even by medical specialists or trained audiologists. Judgments based on responses from patients are more subjective than the experts would like.

Second, no single model of hearing aid can come close to compensating completely for any type of hearing loss.

Third, hearing specialists are handicapped in referring patients to hearing aid dealers by the bewildering array of aids on the market and by the shortage of unbiased technical information about them.

Fourth, hearing specialists lack a reliable means of prescribing a hearing aid with performance characteristics best suited to a patient's needs. It may be possible to specify the patient's requirements in such characteristics as frequency response, gain, maximum power output, and freedom from distortion. But a hearing-aid dealer has little way of relating those specifications to the products at hand. It's likely that if ten people were sent to ten different dealers with the same specifications, they would come back with ten measurably different hearing aids.

That there is a lack of product reliability complicates matters. More than 50 percent of hearing aids tested by the New York League of the Hard-of-Hearing failed to meet manufacturers' advertised specifications. The HEW Task Force said an industrywide standard of quality and performance for hearing aids is "sorely needed" to eliminate wide variations in the performance of aids.

As if there weren't enough medical and technological difficulties in correcting hearing loss, 70 percent of the 600,000 people who buy hearing aids each year further reduce their chances of finding a remedy by failing to enlist professional help initially. According to the HEW Task Force, 85 percent of persons who contact dealers directly are found "capable of being helped" by an aid. In contrast, statistics from the government of Saskatchewan, Canada, show that only 45 percent of persons who contact audiologists in that province are diagnosed as needing a hearing aid.

The United States and Canadian patient groups are presumably similar; they sought help because they couldn't hear well. The Americans, however, were diagnosed by tradespeople interested in selling hearing aids. The Canadians were diagnosed by professionals without a pecuniary interest in aids. Investigations by public-interest groups in New York City and Baltimore came to similar conclusions. They found that in more than 40 percent of the cases studied, dealers recommended the purchase of hearing aids when hearing professionals had already determined that patients could not benefit from the devices.

In addition to commercial motives, the sale of unnecessary hearing aids can be attributed to hard-sell tactics, faulty test equipment, and poor training and regulation of dealers. Beware of any dealer who says than an aid will make hearing absolutely or practically normal or that an aid is essential for "nerve stimulation" to prevent further hearing loss. Those are common but untrue claims. Beware also of the dealer who tests hearing in a less-than-quiet area. A very quiet room is essential for accurate testing.

Extensive testing with calibrated equipment is essential in evaluating a person's need for a hearing aid. Yet only a few of the forty states with licensing laws for dealers require them to use even minimal testing procedures and audiological screening equipment. Fourteen of those states have no system to check the calibration of test devices. In most states that do call for calibration, dealers are required only to file an annual certificate with the licensing boards that their equipment has been calibrated. "Just how well this voluntary reporting system works is unclear," comments a staff study by the Permanent Subcommittee on Investigations of the United States Senate Government Operations Committee.

The basic training for hearing-aid salespersons is a twenty-week home-study course offered by the National Hearing Aid Society (NHAS), the dealers' association. That's the course leading to the designation Certified Hearing Aid Audiologist. The Senate Permanent Subcommittee on Investigations asked several committees of hearing professionals, mainly otologists and audiologists, to evaluate the content of the NHAS home-study course. The experts characterized the course as "inadequate," "inaccurate," and even "potentially dangerous." (The NHAS announced a new, more detailed, college-based training program for dealers in 1975, but the NHAS won't compel attendance or expel members who don't sign up.) The HEW Task Force said that the NHAS home-study course and subsequent examination "do not include any evaluation of the dealer's practical skills in testing and fitting hearing aids, nor of the dealer's ability to communicate with and counsel the hearing impaired."

State regulation of hearing-aid dealers is, at best, uneven. Forty states now have licensure laws for dealers, but most of them are modeled on a bill proposed by the industry. Only four—Hawaii, Minnesota, New York, and Vermont—require that a person see a doctor or audiologist before buying a hearing aid. Nearly 50 percent of state-licensed dealers were not required to take an examination for the certification. They were "grandfathered" into licenses by virtue of their business activity before the law was passed. Only seven states require applicants for licensure to have had training other than apprenticeship under a licensed dealer. Virginia alone requires an applicant to complete a college-level course.

The NHAS and the hearing-aid manufacturers rely on state licensing agencies to police dealers. But few of the states employ full-time professional staff members for this purpose. The budgets for licensing boards are often minuscule or nonexistent. In thirty-five states, dealers either outnumber the other board members or make up at least one-half the panel, and a number of boards rarely transact business. The staff study of the Senate Permanent Subcommittee on Investigations reached this conclusion: "Most state licensing agencies are controlled by dealers—many of whom have been grandfathered into licensure. These dealers are often responsible for the drafting of loophole-ridden laws in the first place. Once on the board, these dealers frequently band together to frustrate consumer members."

The Senate Permanent Subcommittee on Investigations, at the request of Senator Charles H. Percy of Illinois, in 1975 examined state licensing and training requirements for hearing-aid dealers. Often, the boards seemed to work harder to protect dealers from criticism than to protect consumers from injustices. In the case of Kentucky, the study produced evidence that certain dealer members of the licensing board used that membership to advance personal interests.

Kentucky is one of the many states that allow grand-fathering, a practice that rests on the notion that experience equals competence. One person grandfathered into a Kentucky license was the son of Charles N. Stone, then chairman of the licensing board. The son, Michael Stone, was nineteen when he applied for a license. He stated on his application that he was fourteen when he began working in his father's store. Grandfathering is a dubious practice at best; applied to a teenager, it's ludicrous.

The Senate study also cited an incident involving a Kentucky board member, Marion Roberts, also a hearing-aid dealer. Roberts was asked by a consumer member of the board about his reasons for sponsoring a particular man who applied for a license and about whether he had supervised the man's work for six months, as required by law. According to the other board member, Roberts "replied that the man owed him $4,000 and he must get it back, so he was going to sign an affidavit swearing that he had sponsored the man for six months." A third board member, Norma Jean Phillips, confirmed the story, adding in an affidavit that Roberts told her the applicant was "not of good moral character." (Roberts denied Ms. Phillips's recollection of their conversation.)

Roberts, along with four other dealer-members of the board, including chairman Stone, were involved in a third incident that came to the Senate investigators' attention. In January 1974, the five board members organized the Kentucky College of Otometry, later renamed the National College of Otometry. The college's catalogue detailed a five-year course of study, at $500 per semester, leading to a Doctor of Otometry degree. The five state board members were listed as "regents," and the college's address was the same as Roberts's dealership in Richmond, Ky.

At its meeting in November 1974, the board heard a suggestion from member Larry J. Naiser, one of the college's regents, that the board officially commend the college. A formal motion to approve the college was neither offered nor voted upon. Yet shortly afterward, Marion Roberts wrote to hearing-aid dealers around the state, inviting them to a seminar at the college's campus at which "certified otometrist" wall plaques would be issued to those who paid the $60 attendance fee. The letter began: "Our State licensing board has approved the 'National College of Otometry' and are [sic] in the process of writing the College of Otometry a commendation."

The Kentucky attorney general filed suit the following April against the National College of Otometry and two of its regents, including Roberts, for false and misleading practices. The suit charged that the institution was not a duly accredited college and had no authority to issue a doctoral degree. The terms otometry and otometrist are reserved for professional audiologists, the suit alleged. The challenged representations, according to the suit, "will mislead and cause consumers to seek advice, assistance, and treatment related to hearing and disorders of hearing from recipients of the defendants' otometry degree and cause such consumers to part with substantial sums of money, and risk serious and irreparable harm and damage to their hearing and psychological health."

In May 1975, the defendants agreed to an order prohibiting the use of the words otometry and otometrist and prohibiting any representation that the state board had approved the college. In accordance with the conditions of the order, Marion Roberts wrote to dealers who had attended the conference, offering refunds on the $60 paid for the certified otometrist plaques. He explained that "the Certificate issued to you at our November 1974 Conference is to be considered valueless, is not to be displayed, and could be considered a violation of the Kentucky Consumer Protection Act."

Hearings before the Senate Subcommittee on Consumer Interests of the Elderly provided case histories of the dangers of purchasing a hearing aid without prior medical consultation. Among them were examples offered by the Minnesota Public Interest Research Group:

A sixty-eight-year-old stroke victim with expressive aphasia (a loss of the ability to speak) was sold two aids although he had normal hearing.

A forty-four-year-old man with conductive hearing loss was sold two hearing aids. When he finally saw a physician, surgery restored him to almost normal hearing.

A sixty-eight-year-old man was tested and fitted by a dealer with an in-the-ear hearing aid too weak to compensate for his loss. Professional examinations later found the aid to be completely inadequate and a different aid was prescribed.

Certainly, not all hearing aid dealers are guilty of such practices. Many, it should be acknowledged, have extensive practical experience with hearing problems. And many more are sincerely interested in helping people hear better. The HEW Task Force said that "the various services (e.g., fitting an aid, pre- and post-paid counseling, and repairs) provided by these specialists are regarded by many of the hard-of-hearing as indispensable to their welfare." Still, CU believes that the prospective purchaser of a hearing aid would be wise to view dealers as tradespeople who can be helpful in explaining the workings of and problems associated with hearing aids, but not as professionals competent to diagnose and solve a hearing problem.

So, when you walk into a hearing-aid dealer's store, you'll be there just as a customer, not as a patient or examinee. If you've followed the steps CU has outlined, you'll take with you specific instructions from an otologist or audiologist (although, as we have explained, the instructions may not always be readily interpretable into the name of a specific model). You don't need any further evaluations or a sales pitch. But you could get a price break in return for not using the dealer's testing and evaluation services. Some dealers can be persuaded to give a discount, so ask for one.

The dealer will probably take an impression of your ear canal to make an earpiece if one has not already been provided by the audiologist. A charge of $15 or $20 extra is common for that. And the dealer can be quite helpful in showing you how to operate and take care of the aid.

You should insist that the aid be bought on a trial basis only. Reputable dealers will rent you the aid for a month at the rate of about $1 a day. If you aren't satisfied, they'll take it back and, if you buy the aid, they'll deduct the rental fee from the price. The FTC has proposed a new regulation that would, in effect, make the thirty-day rental offer mandatory for all dealers, except when specific brand-and-model aids are prescribed by otologists or audiologists. (CU has commented to the FTC that the distinction between prescribed aids and unprescribed aids is unfair because buyers of both types run a risk of getting an aid not right for them.) During the thirty-day trial period, you should return to the otologist or audiologist to find out whether the aid is working properly. Unless something is obviously wrong, try your new aid the full month to become accustomed to it. If you can't get used to it, you may decide that you want to seek rehabilitative help.

Dealers defend their high markups in terms of the time they devote to testing, fitting, and following the progress of their customers. In our view, however, testing is a job for otologists and audiologists.* And a patient experiencing difficulty in adjusting to a hearing aid is better served by professional advice, not advice from a dealer. As for fitting the earpiece, dealers often charge extra for that anyway.

Most dealers, in effect, force customers to buy a whole package of services. The HEW Task Force has proposed changing that by "unbundling" the dealer's bill—that is, separating the cost of services from the cost of the hearing aid, thus permitting buyers to pay only for those services they need. The Task Force recommended that all state licensure and registration laws for hearing-aid dealers contain a requirement for unbundled, itemized bills. CU has suggested to the FTC that it include the unbundling requirement in a new trade regulation under consideration for the hearing-aid industry. We did so because the reform would be quicker, surer, and more uniform under federal, rather than state, jurisdiction.

But there is a possibility that much the same kind of reform can be accomplished at the commercial level. A star example is Master Plan Service Co. of Minneapolis, which now has franchises in nineteen cities. Master Plan attempts to carry as many hearing-aid lines as possible, de-

*In April 1976 the United States Food and Drug Administration proposed rules requiring hearing-aid dealers to direct customers to physicians for a medical examination before selling them an aid. But the proposed rules contain a massive loophole. Adult customers, except under certain limited circumstances, can sign a paper waiving the medical examination when purchasing a hearing aid. Dealers in pursuit of a fast sale will be tempted to push the waiver, not the medical examination.

spite resistance from manufacturers who prefer exclusive or limited-line dealerships. Master Plan does little advertising and no prospecting for clients. It accepts orders only on referral from otologists and audiologists, and it does no testing or evaluation of patients. It just sells and services prescribed aids at a cost of $150 or more below list price. In our view, the Master Plan approach properly divides responsibility between the professional and trade members of the hearing-aid delivery system.

Financial assistance from the government is limited. Medicaid programs in twenty-six states,* Guam, and the Virgin Islands offer assistance to certain categories of people who cannot afford to buy a hearing aid. The program covers diagnosis of the hearing problem and purchase of the aid. But the criteria for determining need are fairly restrictive.

The Medicare program for the elderly provides assistance only for diagnosis leading to ear surgery—not for diagnosis calling for a hearing aid nor for purchase of the aid itself.

The Federal Rehabilitation Services Administration, working through state departments of vocational rehabilitation, assists people whose hearing problems handicap employment. (Homemaking is often viewed as an eligible form of employment.) Information can be obtained from your state vocational rehabilitation agency. General information on deafness and hearing and speech impairment can be obtained from the Office of Deafness and Communications Disorders, Rehabilitation Services Administration,

*California, Connecticut, Illinois, Indiana, Iowa, Kansas, Louisiana, Massachusetts, Minnesota, Montana, Nebraska, Nevada, New Hampshire, New Jersey, New Mexico, New York, North Dakota, Ohio, Oregon, Rhode Island, Utah, Virginia, Vermont, Washington, West Virginia, and Wisconsin.

Office of Human Development, Department of Health, Education, and Welfare, Washington, D.C. 20201.

Help for children is provided through the federal Maternal and Child Health Service. The program is administered through state health departments or state crippled-children's services, which should be contacted for information. The children's service arranges for diagnostic work and hearing aids at no cost or at reduced prices, depending on need.

Veterans can obtain free diagnostic services and hearing aids from the Veterans Administration. Assistance is usually limited to veterans whose hearing losses are service-connected or to patients in VA hospitals.

The American Speech and Hearing Association's *Guide to Clinical Services in Speech Pathology and Audiology* lists more than 1,882 sources of speech and hearing clinical services, many of which have been accredited by ASHA. The full guide costs $6 ($8 for nonmembers), but a list of facilities in your area is available free on request. Also free is a useful ASHA pamphlet entitled *Hearing Impairment and the Audiologist*. Write to the American Speech and Hearing Association, 9030 Old Georgetown Road, Washington, D.C. 20014.

UNDERSTANDING THE VA RATINGS

The Veterans Administration tests only about 20 to 25 percent of the hearing aids on the market. Still, for the 1976 model year, it tested more than a hundred hearing aids—far more than CU could possibly test in a program of our own. Our summary of the VA ratings is meant primarily for otologists and audiologists. As in 1971, CU endorses the

VA's view that the selection of an aid should not be made solely by studying its ratings but rather requires professional guidance, as described earlier in this report.

The VA invites manufacturers to enter aids of their choice for the testing program. The aids submitted must be standard, currently available production models. VA representatives pick three random samples of each aid from the manufacturers' stock. Those samples are tested for the VA by the Sound Section of the Institute of Basic Standards at the National Bureau of Standards, and the Bicommunications Laboratory at the University of Maryland.

Raw data from the tests are analyzed by the VA's Auditory Research Laboratory and, in most cases, are converted into a performance score. The VA also considers cost, dividing the cost of an aid (usually a discounted price) by the performance score to determine lowest cost per point of quality. Administration contracts are awarded on the basis of superior performance scores, lowest cost per quality point, and particular characteristics needed for clinical reasons. In addition, the VA considers the previous year's record of repair service.

As in the past, our introduction here to the VA ratings is but a brief summary of the tests from which they were derived. One can obtain the complete test report, *Handbook of Hearing Aid Measurement, 1976,* from the Superintendent of Documents, United States Government Printing Office, Washington, D.C. 20402, for $5.50.

This 1976 report goes into detail about the various test methods used, including those for many specialized aids. Tests included measurements of frequency response, gain, maximum power output, battery current drain, harmonic distortion, signal-to-noise ratio, and hum immunity. The VA also checked to see whether the aids are clinically acceptable—that is, whether they're easy to wear and to use.

The measurements for each electronic characteristic were scored and weighted according to criteria developed by the VA to produce an overall performance score. A score of 100 is average for an aid within its category. Scores above and below this point represent proportionately better or worse aids. Most of the test data used to score the aids can be read directly from the government report. In the ratings that follow, the technical information is limited to average gain, average maximum power output, and overall performance score.

In 1971, we calculated and published the Index of Effectiveness (I of E), a factor that received heaviest weighting in the VA's scoring scheme. But it had to be extrapolated from various secondary data. And since the VA is currently reevaluating and modifying its hearing aid evaluation criteria, CU is unable to provide the I of E. Also, the VA's scoring scheme may be modified for aids with special characteristics or not computed at all. In 1976, for example, the VA did not compute performance scores for high-frequency-emphasis, in-the-ear, CROS, and BI-CROS aids.

The VA has reported which aids it selected for contract or, in the case of those not selected, which aids nonetheless scored in the top 25 percent of their category. In the ratings, which follow, such models are indicated by black dots.

VETERANS ADMINISTRATION RATINGS OF HEARING AIDS

Listed by categories. Models with standard acoustic characteristics are categorized by power: strong, moderate, and mild. Within power categories, listed in order of decreasing performance score (with 100 as average). Models with unique characteristics are categorized by specialty and, except as noted, are listed in order of decreasing performance score. Performance scores were not computed by the VA for CROS, BICROS, high-frequency-emphasis, and in-the-ear aids. Models preceded by a black dot have been selected for purchase by the VA and/or scored in the top 25 percent of their category. All figures are rounded to the nearest whole number. Prices are given when available from manufacturers and are list, as stated by them, rounded to the nearest dollar.

Described by type: body (on-the-body), over ear (behind or over-the-ear), eyeglass, and in-the-ear. Except as noted, average gain is the amplification in decibels (dB) as computed by the VA over the frequency range of 500 to 2,000 Hz.; for high-frequency-emphasis aids, gain was computed over the range of 1,000 to 2,000 Hz. Average maximum power output (the amplification cut-off point) is in dB computed over the speech spectrum range.

STRONG-POWER MODELS

Brand and model	Type	Average gain	Average maximum power output	Perfor- mance score
●OTICON 375 PPX (Oticon Corp., Union, N.J.), $415.	Body	59	131	121
●TELEX 70 (Telex Communications, Inc., Minneapolis)	Body	61	133	113
●ZENITH VOCALIZER III (Zenith Hearing Instrument Corp., Chicago), $335.	Body	63	135	97
RADIOEAR 980 (Radioear Corp., Cannonsburg, Pa.)	Body	63	135	96
●AUDIVOX 115X11 (Air) (Audivox Hearing Aids, Newton, Mass.), $405.	Over ear	59	130	87
●LEHR OMNITON 115F (Lehr Instrument Corp., Huntington Station, N.Y.)	Body	62	135	63
DANAVOX 727 PPE (Danavox, Inc., Minneapolis)	Body	62	133	52

Brand and model	Type	Average gain	Average maximum power output	Performance score
ACOUSTICON A770 Gold (HP receiver) (Acousticon Systems Corp., Danbury, Conn.)	Body	67	139	38
●SONOTONE 670 BX (Sonotone Corp., Elmsford, N.Y.)	Body	72	142	33

MODERATE-POWER MODELS

Brand and model	Type	Average gain	Average maximum power output	Performance score
●ZENITH PACE EPII (Zenith Hearing Instrument Corp.), $395.	Over ear	52	127	150
●OTICON S-11-V (Oticon Corp.), $425.	Eyeglass	44	118	142
●OTICON E-11-V (Oticon Corp.), $420.	Over ear	45	118	132
●AUDIOTONE A-24D (Audiotone Div., Royal Industries, Phoenix)	Over ear	45	119	130
●LEHR OPTICA 6 (Lehr Instrument Corp.), $375.	Eyeglass	47	121	123
●SONOTONE 40-6 (Sonotone Corp.)	Eyeglass	51	123	122
●RADIOEAR 1050 (Radioear Corp.)	Over ear	54	127	120
●SONOTONE 77-S (Sonotone Corp.)	Over ear	55	124	118
●LEHR STAR 6F (Lehr Instrument Corp.), $395.	Over ear	55	127	116
TELEX 334 RD (Telex Communications, Inc.)Ⓐ	Over ear	64	127	116
WIDEX A2-T (Widex Hearing Aid Co., Long Island City, N.Y.)	Over ear	53	127	115
OTICON E-18-P (Oticon Corp.), $455.	Over ear	56	130	113

Brand and model	Type	Average gain	Average maximum power output	Performance score
AUDIOTONE A-24 (Audiotone Div., Royal Industries)	Over ear	46	119	112
VICON 124 (Vicon Instrument Co., Colorado Springs, Colo.)	Over ear	45	118	112
AUDIOTONE A-20 (Audiotone Div., Royal Industries)	Over ear	45	121	108
QUALITONE TPF (Qualitone, Inc., Minneapolis), $355.	Over ear	53	126	107
QUALITONE TSP (Qualitone, Inc.), $370.	Over ear	55	129	103
AUDIVOX 111 Spectacular, RD response (Audivox Hearing Aids), $390.	Eyeglass	54	128	102
VICON 150 (Vicon Instrument Co.)	Over ear	54	127	102
REXTON 4134 (Starkey Labs, Inc., Eden Praine, Minn.)	Body	50	124	101
AUDIOTONE A-25 (Audiotone Div., Royal Industries)	Over ear	44	120	100
AUDIOTONE A-23 (Audiotone Div., Royal Industries)	Over ear	55	128	99
RADIOEAR 1040 (Radioear Corp.)	Eyeglass	55	127	98
Danavox 695 PPE (Danavox, Inc.)	Over ear	55	127	97
NORTH AMERICAN PHILIPS HP8276E (North American Philips Corp., NYC), $414.	Over ear	55	128	97
DAHLBERG HT 1233 (Dahlberg Electronics, Inc., Golden Valley, Minn.)	Over ear	55	128	96
VICON 123 (Vicon Instrument Co.)	Over ear	48	119	93
OTICON 380 SI (Oticon Corp.), $250.	Body	55	125	89
DAHLBERG RP 2528 (Dahlberg Electronics, Inc.)	Over ear	52	125	85
WIDEX 77 (Widex Hearing Aid Co.)	Over ear	47	119	85
REXTON 4136 (Starkey Labs, Inc.)🅱	Over ear	52	124	83

Brand and model	Type	Average gain	Average maximum power output	Performance score
VICON M-8 (Vicon Instrument Co.)	Body	54	131	81
FIDELITY F-339 (Fidelity Electronics, Ltd., Chicago), $390.	Body	57	128	78
SIEMENS 24PP PC (Siemens Corp., Union, N.J.), $460.	Over ear	56	128	78
DANAVOX 735-S (Danavox, Inc.)	Over ear	48	121	77
FIDELITY F-39 (Fidelity Electronics, Ltd.), $490	Over ear	56	128	75
●DAHLBERG HF-1250 (Dahlberg Electronics, Inc.)	Eyeglass	58	129	74
OTARION TONETTE (Otarion Electronics, Inc., Ossining, N.Y.)	Over ear	44	118	56
●ZENITH AWARD (Zenith Hearing Instrument Corp.), $99.	Body	—	—	—

MILD-POWER MODELS

Brand and model	Type	Average gain	Average maximum power output	Performance score
●QUALITONE UFO (Qualitone, Inc.), $368.	Over ear	31	112	149
●OTICON E-16-U (Oticon Corp.), $299.	Over ear	39	113	138
●NORTH AMERICAN PHILIPS HP8252 (North American Philips Corp.), $285.	Over ear	37	112	126
●QUALITONE 155 (Qualitone, Inc.), $360.	Over ear	39	121	125
●REXTON 4112 (Starkey Labs, Inc.) Ⓒ	Over ear	35	114	120
●AUDIVOX 37 Micronic (Audivox Hearing Aids), $285.	Eyeglass	41	113	118

Ⓐ *According to the company, this model has been discontinued.*
Ⓑ *Directional.* Ⓒ *Compression.* Ⓓ *Option for directional.*
Ⓔ *According to the company, this model has been replaced by model DH.* Ⓕ *BICROS.* Ⓖ *CROS.*

Brand and model	Type	Average gain	Average maximum power output	Performance score
ACOUSTICON A-690 w/"A" tone control, —2 (Acousticon Systems Corp.)	Over ear	36	113	113
DANAVOX 745 V (Danavox, Inc.)	Over ear	44	118	112
LEHR STAR 44 (Lehr Instrument Corp.)	Over ear	40	114	112
DAHLBERG RL 2527 (Dahlberg Electronics, Inc.)	Over ear	38	113	109
TELEX 334 (Telex Communications, Inc.)	Over ear	37	110	96
ACOUSTICON A-650R (Acousticon Systems Corp.)	Over ear	39	113	93
AUDIVOX 123 Bi-Focal, RD response (Audivox Hearing Aids), $405. D	Eyeglass	39	113	81
DAHLBERG PA 2526 (Dahlberg Electronics, Inc.)	Over ear	40	114	81
ACOUSTICON A-465 SSR (Acousticon Systems Corp.)	In ear	29	109	—
OTARION LISTENETTE (Otarion Electronics, Inc.)	In ear	40	114	—

COMPRESSION MODELS

Brand and model	Type	Average gain	Average maximum power output	Performance score
•OTICON 565 SZ LDC (Oticon Corp.) A	Over ear	30	106	143
•VICON 159 (Vicon Instrument Co.) B	Over ear	36	112	120
•H-C 527SE with N transducer (H-C Electronics, Inc., Mill Valley, Calif.), $255.	Body	64	122	119
•NORTH AMERICAN PHILIPS HP8274 (North American Philips Corp.), $438.	Over ear	45	117	119
H-C 527L with N transducer (H-C Electronics, Inc.), $413.	Body	64	123	114
•QUALITONE CSD (Qualitone, Inc.), $355. B	Over ear	30	106	113
FIDELITY F-37 (Fidelity Electronics, Ltd.), $430.	Over ear	43	115	109

Brand and model	Type	Average gain	Average maximum power output	Performance score
ZENITH COMMAND 100 (Zenith Hearing Instrument Corp.), $395.	Over ear	33	106	108
●H-C 527L with W transducer (H-C Electronics, Inc.), $413.	Body	62	120	94
SIEMENS 32D-AGC (Siemens Corp.), $435. Ⓑ	Over ear	52	116	93
SIEMENS 22-AVC (Siemens Corp.), $428.	Over ear	38	110	92
●H-C 527SE with W transducer (H-C Electronics, Inc.), $255.	Body	62	119	91
H-C 527L with PP transducer (H-C Electronics, Inc.), $413.	Body	71	129	82
H-C 527SE with PP transducer (H-C Electronics, Inc.), $255.	Body	70	128	77
RADIOEAR 1030 (Radioear Corp.) Ⓑ	Over ear	50	121	75
NORTH AMERICAN PHILIPS HP8275 (North American Philips Corp.), $438.	Over ear	36	108	27
H-C 527PE (H-C Electronics, Inc.)	Body	—	—	—
SHALAKO 1421 (Shalako International, Scottsdale, Ariz.)	Over ear	23	107	—
SHALAKO 1511 (Shalako International)	Body	18	112	—

DIRECTIONAL MODELS

Brand and model	Type	Average gain	Average maximum power output	Performance score
●REXTON 4137 (Starkey Labs, Inc.)	Over ear	38	115	133
●QUALITONE CSD (Qualitone, Inc.), $355. Ⓒ	Over ear	30	106	132
●VICON 159 (Vicon Instrument Co.) Ⓒ	Over ear	36	112	131

Ⓐ *According to the company, this model has been discontinued.*
Ⓑ *Directional.* Ⓒ *Compression.* Ⓓ *Option for directional.*
Ⓔ *According to the company, this model has been replaced by model DH.* Ⓕ *BICROS.* Ⓖ *CROS.*

Brand and model	Type	Average gain	Average maximum power output	Performance score
●NORTH AMERICAN PHILIPS HP8283E (North American Philips Corp.), $405.	Over ear	47	120	130
●LEHR STAR 6 AVCD (Lehr Instrument Corp.)	Over ear	42	120	114
●ZENITH ROYAL D (Zenith Hearing Instrument Corp.), $425.	Over ear	53	126	113
●NORTH AMERICAN PHILIPS HP8288E (North American Philips Corp.), $405.	Over ear	43	115	110
AUDIOTONE A-27 (Audiotone Div., Royal Industries)	Over ear	45	127	106
DANAVOX 735 DS (Danavox, Inc.)	Over ear	45	120	104
SIEMENS 32 D-AGC (Siemens Corp.), $435. Ⓒ	Over ear	52	116	99
SIEMENS 34D-SL (Siemens Corp.), $460.	Over ear	53	127	94
ACOUSTICON A-690 D (Acousticon Systems Corp.)	Over ear	48	120	89
VICON 158 (Vicon Instrument Co.)	Over ear	52	127	85
RADIOEAR 1030 (Radioear Corp.) Ⓒ	Over ear	50	121	75
FIDELITY F-58D (Fidelity Electronics, Ltd.), $490.	Over ear	43	116	72
MAICO CQ (Maico Hearing Instruments, Minneapolis) Ⓔ	Over ear	40	113	69
TELEX 33D (Telex Communications, Inc.)	Over ear	52	126	46

HIGH-FREQUENCY-EMPHASIS MODELS

■ *The VA did not compute performance scores for the following models. Listed in order of decreasing gain.*

LEHR OPTICA 6 BIFROS (Lehr Instrument Corp.), $705.	Special eyeglass	32	124	—
●NORTH AMERICAN PHILIPS HP8269 (North American Philips Corp.), $405.	Over ear	31	120	—

Brand and model	Type	Average gain	Average maximum power output	Performance score
AUDIOVOX 101 CYCLORAMIC II, DGD response (Audiovox Hearing Aids), $345.	Over ear	26	117	—
ACOUSTICON A-650 HP (Acousticon Systems Corp.)	Over ear	25	119	—
MAICO DE (Maico Hearing Instruments)	Over ear	24	118	—
SIEMENS 26H (Siemens Corp.), $421.	Over ear	24	123	—
WIDEX 85 (Widex Hearing Aid Co.)	Over ear	24	122	—
DAHLBERG NP2521 (Dahlberg Electronics, Inc.)Ⓑ	Over ear	20	121	—
SONOTONE 50-2 (Sonotone Corp.)	Eyeglass	19	119	—
ZENITH DOVER C (Zenith Hearing Instrument (Corp.), $375.	Over ear	17	121	—
•TELEX 331 H (Telex Communications, Inc.)	Over ear	15	119	—
DANAVOX 743 UN (Danavox, Inc.)	Over ear	14	117	—
LEHR STAR 6H (Lehr Instrument Corp.), $395.	Over ear	13	121	—
•AUDIOTONE A-20 P-5 (Audiotone Div., Royal Industries)	Over ear	12	125	—

CROS AND BICROS MODELS

■ *The VA did not compute performance scores for the following models. Listed in order of decreasing gain; the gain reported for CRO aids was measured at 2,000 Hz; for BICROS aids, 1,000 Hz.*

TELEX 334 BC (Telex Communications, Inc.)Ⓐ Ⓕ	Over ear	61	127	—

Ⓐ *According to the company, this model has been discontinued.*
Ⓑ *Directional.* Ⓒ *Compression.* Ⓓ *Option for directional.*
Ⓔ *According to the company, this model has been replaced by model DH.* Ⓕ *BICROS.* Ⓖ *CROS.*

Brand and model	Type	Average gain	Average maximum power output	Performance score
TELEX 334 SC (Telex Communications, Inc.) Ⓐ Ⓖ	Over ear	59	129	—
●QUALITONE TSPNB (Qualitone, Inc.), $445. Ⓕ	Eyeglass	58	130	—
SIEMENS 24E SL-PC (Siemens Corp.), $439. Ⓕ	Over ear	58	129	—
●DAHLBERG HG 1250 (Dahlberg Electronics, Inc.) Ⓕ	Eyeglass	56	128	—
OTICON S11V (Oticon Corp.), $425. Ⓖ	Eyeglass	55	119	—
●RADIOEAR 1040 (Radioear Corp.) Ⓕ	Eyeglass	51	127	—
SONOTONE 35 AX (Sonotone Corp.) Ⓕ	Eyeglass	51	123	—
OTARION X-102 (Otarion Electronics, Inc.) Ⓕ	Eyeglass	49	120	—
VICON OE-124 (Vicon Instrument Co.) Ⓖ	Over ear	49	123	—
VIENNATONE ALPC/C (Viennatone of America, Inc., Chicago) Ⓖ	Eyeglass	49	117	—
BELTONE SONATA STANDARD (Beltone Electronics Corp., Chicago) Ⓖ	Over ear	47	117	—
RADIOEAR 1010 (Radioear Corp.) Ⓖ	Eyeglass	47	120	—
●SIEMENS H28E MP HF (Siemens Corp.), $421. Ⓖ	Over ear	47	117	—
ACOUSTICON 1001 (Acousticon Systems Corp.) Ⓖ	Eyeglass	46	118	—
AUDIVOX 123C (Audivox Hearing Aids), $450. Ⓖ	Eyeglass	46	115	—
●DAHLBERG JC1254 (Dahlberg Electronics, Inc.) Ⓖ	Eyeglass	46	118	—
FIDELITY F52C (Fidelity Electronics, Ltd.), $490. Ⓖ	Over ear	45	113	—
OTICON 850S (Oticon Corp.) Ⓕ	Eyeglass	45	120	—
●AUDIOTONE A 24 (Audiotone Div., Royal Industries) Ⓕ	Over ear	44	118	—

Brand and model	Type	Average gain	Average maximum power output	Performance score
SONOTONE 35 AZ (Sonotone Corp.) Ⓖ	Eyeglass	44	125	—
VICON OE-124 (Vicon Instrument Co.) Ⓕ	Over ear	43	119	—
AUDIOTONE A24 (Audiotone Div., Royal Industries) Ⓖ	Over ear	42	120	—
AUDIVOX 123BC (Audivox Hearing Aids), $480. Ⓕ	Eyeglass	42	116	—
BELTONE ARIA STANDARD (Beltone Electronics Corp.) Ⓖ	Over ear	42	110	—
ACOUSTICON 1001 (Acousticon Systems Corp.) Ⓕ	Eyeglass	38	118	—
FIDELITY F490BC (Fidelity Electronics, Ltd.), $490. Ⓕ	Eyeglass	35	119	—
QUALITONE SNEC (Qualitone, Inc.), $400. Ⓖ	Eyeglass	34	123	—
VIENNATONE ALPC/BC (Viennatone of America, Inc.) Ⓕ	Eyeglass	34	120	—
OTARION X-101 (Otarion Electronics, Inc.) Ⓖ	Eyeglass	32	117	—
●ZENITH CROS Zenith Hearing Instrument Corp.), $390. Ⓖ	Eyeglass	29	121	—

SPECIAL MODEL

(Binaural phase related. Different frequency response on each side.)

ZENITH BIPHASIC Zenith Hearing Instrument Corp.), $690.	Eyeglass	—	—	—

Ⓐ *According to the company, this model has been discontinued.*
Ⓑ *Directional.* Ⓒ *Compression.* Ⓓ *Option for directional.*
Ⓔ *According to the company, this model has been replaced by model DH.* Ⓕ *BICROS.* Ⓖ *CROS.*

How to Find a Good Auto Mechanic

From start to finish—from the friendly smile of the service manager to the final bill—getting a car fixed can be tricky business. If the service manager pulls down a percentage of each order written, as is often the case, there's little incentive to do work as inexpensively as possible. And the labor charge included in the final bill is probably based on the number of hours a manual says it takes to do the job, even if a mechanic actually did the work in less time. In between can lie incompetence, long delays, unrealistically low estimates, and overcharges for parts or charges for parts not used.

The car owner with little knowledge of what goes on under the hood thus faces some perplexing decisions. A strange noise can mean a ten-minute adjustment, or it can indicate the need for several hundred dollars in engine repairs. A car can run poorly because a wire is loose or because a major component has failed. The mechanic who usually makes these decisions for the car owner may be one who is competent or incompetent, honest or dishonest.

Statistics on the quality of auto repairs are not reassuring. In 1972, the St. Louis diagnostic clinic of the Automobile Club of Missouri rechecked more than a thousand cars repaired by auto mechanics. The clinic found that 28.7 percent of the repairs were done unsatisfactorily or, unknown to the car owner, not at all. The average repair bill for the incompetent or fraudulent work was $127. In 1974 the clinic did a new survey. This time 37.7 percent of the repairs were done badly or not at all, and the average repair bill came to $148.

In only four cities in the United States can consumers get impartial guidance. The Missouri American Automobile Association (AAA) diagnostic clinics in St. Louis and Kansas City will tell you what repairs your car needs and then check afterward on whether the repairs were done properly. The clinics will not recommend a mechanic, however.

The AAA is recommending specific repair shops in Washington, D.C., and Orlando, Fla., as part of a pilot project. Before approving a facility, AAA inspectors will fill out an elaborate report on the appearance of the shop, its equipment, the qualifications of the mechanics, and its reputation with consumer agencies and randomly selected customers. In return for AAA approval, the shop must offer a written estimate and get the customer's authorization for any work that exceeds that estimate by 10 percent, make available parts that were replaced, and guarantee the service work for 90 days or 4,000 miles.

Perhaps most important, there's also a grievance procedure. AAA inspectors will investigate complaints and, if necessary, order the shop to do the repair over or refund the money. The Washington program started in October 1975; by the end of the year there were already a half-dozen rulings against the approved garages, a good showing.

CU, of course, can't judge the quality of repairs done by the approved shops. But, because of safeguards like the guarantee and the grievance procedure, we'd suggest that readers who live near Washington or Orlando seek out repair shops recommended by the AAA.

The vast majority of American car owners, of course, must choose a mechanic without any sort of professional guidance. CU has consulted experts in the field and assembled some suggestions that might prove helpful in making the choice. We present them here in full knowledge that competence doesn't guarantee honesty nor honesty competence. But we also present these suggestions in the belief that, while not foolproof, they can increase your chances of getting decent work at a fair price.

If you buy a new car, don't feel you're tied to that dealer's shop. Only the dealer from whom you bought the car or another dealer who handles the same model is authorized to perform repairs under warranty. But you may take your car anywhere for the routine maintenance prescribed in the owner's manual. Just be sure you keep copies of the itemized bills as evidence that problems covered by the warranty didn't result from any failure on your part to maintain the car.

Of course, you may well want the dealer's shop to do all work on the car while it's still new, particularly if you expect to put the car in the condition it should have been in when delivered. But thereafter consider the pros and cons of dealership maintenance and repair.

A dealer has the advantage of close contact with the factory. The dealership receives all service bulletins and may often get briefings about complex repair problems. The mechanics who work at the dealer's shop tend to become expert at servicing and repairing the models sold there. And a dealer may care about keeping customers happy, hoping for repeat new-car sales. Because of factory requirements, and because a dealership tends to be a high-capital operation, the shop may well be equipped with useful and expensive repair and diagnostic equipment not found at every corner service station.

There are problems. The person writing the service order may earn a commission on repairs. So inexpensive repairs mean less money for the service writer than if the work were done in an expensive way (and if the repairs are not under warranty). Auto manufacturers offer service departments a relatively low return on warranty work. To make up for that, dealers' shops tend to charge fancy fees for routine service and for nonwarranty work. Dealer shops usually use parts supplied by the auto companies, which tend to be more expensive than other brands of replacement parts. And, of course, it's rarely possible to develop a one-to-one relationship with the mechanic who actually does the work in a dealer's shop, where there's usually an assembly-line atmosphere.

Is the work done at dealerships more satisfactory than work done elsewhere? Available figures are inconclusive. In two studies on whether repairs were done correctly, the Missouri auto club tabulated the percentage of unsatisfactory repairs by type of shop, including auto dealers, mass merchandisers (big retailers and tire companies with service operations), service stations, shops that specialize in brakes, mufflers, or front ends, and independent garages. In 1968, nearly 37 percent of the work done at auto dealers was judged unsatisfactory—the worst showing of any type of repair shop. In 1974, nearly 35 percent of the work done at dealer shops was judged unsatisfactory—but that was the *best* showing that year. (Independent garages did unsatisfactory work 47 percent of the time, according to the 1974 study.)

If you do take your car to a new-car dealer's shop, and if the estimated repair costs are high, visit at least one other dealer or possibly an independent shop for a diagnosis of the problem and an estimate of the repair costs. You can expect to pay something for the diagnosis, but that's the only way to guard against the possibility of an unneeded repair or an unnecessarily expensive repair.

Inspect the repair shop. An efficient shop is almost certain to be busy, since the reputation of a competent mechanic, like that of a good chef, tends to get around. If the shop is well run, it will try to get the cars out as quickly as possible rather than holding on to them for days.

Space should be valuable at a good repair facility, since every parking spot can be used for a paying customer. Be wary, therefore, of a shop with old clunkers around gathering dust. Neatness counts. If the floor is littered with junk and grease, figure that a skilled, well-organized mechanic would be reluctant to work there.

Ask about the equipment. As one of the conditions for approving a repair shop, AAA in Washington, D.C., requires that the facility have more than fifty basic pieces of equipment. The list wouldn't help the typical car owner much, however, since it's unlikely that a mechanic would be willing to review all the shop's equipment with a potential customer, explaining what's owned and what's substituted for desirable equipment not owned. Moreover, few customers not themselves mechanics would recognize the equipment when they saw it or understand the necessarily technical discussion.

But the day of the mechanic who relies solely on informed guesswork and experimentation has passed. So you should see that the mechanic who keeps up your car has and uses certain equipment now considered basic.

As a minimum for a proper tune-up, a mechanic must use a dwell-tachometer, a timing light, a compression tester, and a vacuum gauge. Ask about these very common and relatively inexpensive pieces of equipment. If they're not owned or not used, it's likely that a good tune-up will be more a matter of luck than of skill.

When there are engine problems that require diagnosis, a mechanic can figure out the problem inefficiently, by replacing one component after another until things work right, or efficiently with the help of an engine analyzer with an oscilloscope. An engine analyzer is an instrument that gives readings on various elements of engine performance. Give points to a shop that has and uses this diagnostic aid.

One other piece of equipment needed to check the combined effect of various systems on gas mileage and emissions levels is an infrared exhaust gas analyzer. (Some engine analyzers incorporate it.) This is essentially a photoelectric device that reads the constitutents in the exhaust gas; the device can detect malfunctions a mechanic may not find by experimentation.

Look for NIASE certification. A group called the National Institute for Automotive Service Excellence (NIASE), financed largely by auto manufacturers and parts suppliers, sponsors voluntary tests that certify mechanics in any of eight different repair specialties, including engine repair, engine tune-up, brakes, automatic and manual transmissions, and electrical systems. Passing the NIASE tests reflects mechanical ability about as well as passing, a written test could.

By June 1976, 97,343 mechanics had passed one or more of the NIASE tests, which have been given since 1972. Those who pass may wear on their work clothes an NIASE certification patch and additional patches listing each specialty test they've passed. A directory of repair shops that employ NIASE-certified mechanics is available for $1.95 from NIASE, 1825 K Street N.W., Washington, D.C. 20006.

Some caveats about NIASE certification are in order. First, a repair shop with but one mechanic certified in but one specialty can list itself in the directory or advertise, "We employ mechanics certified by NIASE." The mechanic who actually works on your car may never have taken the test—unless you insist that an NIASE mechanic certified in the area of your repair does the job. Second, there is no grievance procedure; you can't get help from NIASE if a mechanic botches the work. Finally, the certification should be taken only for what it is—proof that the mechanic has theoretical competence. "We never pretend that certification will stop a man from being fraudulent," an NIASE spokesman said. "All we're saying is if you go in to have your brakes fixed, and this man is certified in brakes, this man is competent. We can't even guarantee he will do a good job, because his employer might be rushing him or he might have had a fight with his wife."

Patronize only those shops willing to deal fairly. The shop should agree to give you a written estimate and not to exceed that estimate without your authorization for additional work. Don't be talked out of an estimate by a mechanic who can't say what's wrong until the engine is taken apart. In that case you should get a price for the work necessary to make a diagnosis, then the mechanic should call you for authorization with the estimate for the actual repair.

Ask for a written guarantee. A mechanic should be willing to guarantee the work and the parts for 90 days or 4,000 miles, whichever comes first. (Major parts are usually guaranteed for that period by the supplier.) If it's your mechanic who does the major transmission work or an engine overhaul, ask for a guarantee of one year or 12,000 miles. If the mechanic installs a transmission or an engine rebuilt elsewhere, the guarantee will probably be the standard 90 days/4,000 miles offered by the supplier.

It would be nice to find a good repair shop that doesn't use a flat-rate manual—the book that sets arbitrary, and often generous, labor times for each type of repair. But the manual is used almost universally in billing for labor. Some mechanics, however, rely on the manual more as a guide than as a bible and will be reasonable in adjusting labor charges to reflect the time actually spent on the job. If you're shopping among repair shops for a price, this might be a more important criterion than the actual hourly labor rate. It's definitely a subject worth raising with the shop. **Follow a good mechanic, if you find one.** Once you've located a good mechanic, don't change. If that mechanic switches to another shop, move your business there too.

Diagnostic Centers Can Help

A person with little mechanical knowledge and an ominous noise under the hood is usually at the mercy of the mechanic. These days, the quality of mercy is strained.

In December 1975, the *New York Times* visited repair shops in Manhattan and Suffolk County, Long Island, with a car in perfect working order except for a disconnected throttle-valve linkage to the transmission. A clip that held the linkage in place had been removed; the clip was the only part that needed to be replaced. With the linkage disconnected, the car ran but the transmission shifted at wrong speeds, and the gas pedal resisted downward pressure.

The *Times* took the car to twenty-four repair shops, saying only that "something seems to be wrong with the transmission" and that "the car just doesn't seem to be shifting right." Thirteen garages either misdiagnosed the problem completely or performed or recommended expensive and unnecessary work. Seven of the shops offered estimates ranging from $199.95 to $345. Another seven did the necessary repair for under $20, and one did it at no charge.

What the *Times* needed, but couldn't get, was an independent diagnosis from a competent mechanic who had no personal stake in the repair itself. Most diagnostic centers, unfortunately, are connected with repair shops, so you can't tell whether you're getting a real diagnosis or being sold a repair. But in several cities, there's another choice.

In St. Louis and Kansas City, Missouri Automobile Club diagnostic centers use skilled technicians and modern diagnostic equipment to provide a two-hour diagnosis that covers every key area of the car. (Members pay $22.50; nonmembers, $30.50.) The clinics also provide more specific inspections. For example, if a repair shop tells you that you need a new generator and you suspect the trouble might be a loose wire, you can ask the clinic for its opinion before agreeing to the repair. Members are charged at an hourly rate of $22.50 for whatever time it takes, with a $6.50 minimum. A member may then return after the repair is done and find out whether it was done properly; that costs $1.

In San Francisco and San Jose, there are diagnostic clinics run by the California State Automobile Association. Those clinics will do a full diagnosis, but they normally won't look at a specific problem or recheck the car after the repair is made. The charge for most cars is $21 to a member and $26 to a nonmember.

In six cities—Huntsville, Ala., Phoenix and Tucson, Ariz., Washington, D.C., San Juan, P. R., and Chattanooga, Tenn. —the federal government financed experimental diagnostic centers through June 30, 1976. The centers checked cars from model years 1968 through 1973, and the diagnosis was free to customers.

The Phoenix and Tucson centers have closed, but three centers are still operating without federal funding: The Huntsville center is charging $5 per inspection and the University of Alabama agreed to pay for the rest of the center's operating expenses through December 1976. The San Juan center is being funded by the Commonwealth and makes no charges for a diagnosis. The Chattanooga center is charging $10 per inspection, and the city government is picking up the rest of the expenses for operating the center.

Public law allows the federal government to fund three centers through September 30, 1977. The Washington, D.C., center is being fully funded, and the government is considering giving limited funding to two other of the original six centers.

Should Mechanics Be Licensed?

Should individual auto mechanics be licensed? The idea sounds attractive. Licensing could ensure basic competence and, if properly enforced, could reduce the likelihood of fraud.

But attractive as it sounds, the concept of licensing has its problems. Too often, those being licensed gain control of the licensing mechanism and use it to their own advantage rather than the consumer's. In 1973, for instance, 2,149 aspiring general contractors took the Florida Construction Industry Licensing Board's examination—and every one of them flunked. Then, after a flood of protests, the board took a second look at the results and decided that 88 percent had passed.

A second problem with licensing is that it must somehow provide for those already practicing the trade. If they are automatically licensed (under a "grandfather clause") and if the apprenticeship requirements are used to limit the number of people entering the field, the result could be a shortage of trained licensees. That could push up the cost of repairs without guaranteeing more competent work, since it would be years before most mechanics would have taken tests.

To judge the effectiveness of an individual licensing system, the Federal Trade Commission (FTC) in the fall of 1974 took television sets with a burned-out tube to twenty repair shops in each of three areas: California, which registers television-repair shops but doesn't license technicians; Louisiana, which licenses people for television repair; and the District of Columbia, which at the time neither regulated the shops nor licensed the technicians. The FTC found significantly fewer instances of fraud in California (where fraudulent shops can lose their registration and be forced out of business). But there was no difference in the percentage of fraud between licensed Louisiana and unregulated Washington, D.C. Further, the cost of repairs in Louisiana was about 20 percent higher than in the District of Columbia and in California—despite the fact that California has considerably higher wage rates.

Licensing of auto mechanics has been in effect in Ontario, Canada, for more than thirty years. The licensing involves a long apprenticeship, including sessions in school, and an examination given by the government. But the Ontario system has no procedure for taking a license away. It doesn't retest mechanics, doesn't require such good business practices as written estimates, and has no provision for dealing with fraud. In 1973, an Ontario government task force concluded that licensing didn't protect the public and recommended that it be abolished.

In 1976, Hawaii became the first American state to license auto mechanics. The plan automatically "grandfathers in" all mechanics with at least two years' experience. As of July 1, 1976, those who want to work as mechanics must pass a certification test drawn up by Hawaii's Department of Vocational Education to get a license. The grandfathered mechanics will be encouraged to take the test; if 50 percent of the mechanics in an auto repair shop pass the test, the shop can advertise itself as a "certified registered auto-repair shop."

The Hawaii plan poses a number of questions. Does the Department of Vocational Education have the testing skills to devise a certification test? Will most mechanics take the test even though they don't have to, or will grandfathering mean that for decades most of Hawaii's licensed mechanics did nothing but pay $10 to get certified? Will the tests be made difficult enough to be meaningful without restricting the number of new mechanics so severely that prices would be forced up? Will the state actually take away certification on evidence of fraud, or will the license serve as protection against disciplinary action?

State registration of repair shops has been proposed as an alternative to licensing individual mechanics. The state would register repair shops and require them to perform competent repairs. A state agency could investigate consumer complaints with a fleet of unidentified test cars that monitor the performance of the shops. If a shop consistently did shoddy work, it would lose its registration. Repair-shop owners would thus be encouraged to hire skilled mechanics without creating a licensing system that could be manipulated to increase prices.

California has taken a step toward such a system. It currently has a system of mandatory registration of repair shops. The registered shops must follow procedures laid down by the state, such as providing customers with a written estimate and returning removed parts if requested. The shops face suspension or revocation of the registration for violations of the procedures or for fraud.

But California's registration system has a major defect: It does not deal with incompetent work. The state's auto-repair law does forbid "any willful departure from or disregard of accepted trade standards for good and workmanlike repair in any material respect." But the Bureau of Automotive Repair has yet to define standards for specific jobs—what, for example, constitutes a tune-up?—and this section of the California law hasn't been enforced.

The problem, clearly, is not easily solved. The abuses in the auto-repair system intermingle with competence and honesty. Neither of the experiments being tried in Hawaii and California seems likely to solve all of the problems.

Michigan has some regulations governing both mechanics and repair facilities. The state certifies auto mechanics in the eight categories of auto repair set up by the NIASE. In order to be certified, mechanics must take an oral or written examination, given by the state Bureau of Automotive Regulations, testing their ability to diagnose *and* repair motor vehicles.

Michigan law, as of November 1976, also requires motor-vehicle repair facilities to register with the state. In addition, those facilities must prepare an estimate of repair costs, but there is as yet no rule for determining how close to the estimate the actual bill must be. The law also states that replaced parts must be returned to the consumer.

Start a Co-op Shop?

In this report we offer some advice on how to tilt the odds in your favor in the chancy business of choosing a mechanic. And on pages 337-342 you'll find an evaluation of books addressed to those who want to maintain and repair their own cars. But there's a middle road between doing it yourself and the jungle of commercial repair shops.

In a few places across the country consumers have organized auto-repair shops run on the cooperative principle. To join, the consumer pays a one-time membership fee. Members of the co-op make all the business decisions—which mechanics to hire, how much to pay them, and what equipment to buy. If members are dissatisfied with the service, they don't have to change garages. They can replace the mechanics.

One such shop, The Cooperative Garage of Rockland County, West Nyack, N.Y., was organized in November 1975. Within two months, the shop had eighty-five members, each of whom paid $50 to join. It also had one full-time and one part-time mechanic, one full-time bookkeeper (who also filled in as a mechanic when things got busy), and one part-time bookkeeper.

In November 1976, there were over two hundred members. They pay $17.50 an hour for labor. That's no cheaper than the rates many commercial garages in that area charge —but at the co-op, members pay for actual time worked rather than the flat rate charged by most dealers' service shops. Since the mechanics at the co-op are paid a flat salary (rather than one based on the number of jobs performed), they have no incentive to sell customers unnecessary repairs or to rush a job and do careless work.

The co-op members can also save on parts. The co-op buys most parts at wholesale prices and marks them up only 10 percent. Often the mechanics buy parts at local wrecking yards, thus saving members still more money. Or members can bring their own parts, if they prefer.

CU found no shortage of enthusiasm and willingness to sacrifice among those involved in the co-op. During the first two months of its existence, when money was short, the full-time mechanic and bookkeeper drew considerably less than their full salaries. By November 1976, the co-op had three full-time mechanics who earned weekly salaries below the going rate and took turns working on weekends.

There *is* a drawback, however: The co-op's "garage"— a converted dairy—has no car lift. To do work on the undercarriage of a car, a mechanic must use a hydraulic jack, which can be inconvenient and time-consuming. Thus, some extensive repair jobs, such as a muffler replacement, might cost more at the co-op than at a commercial garage, even with the savings for parts. (There is, however, a stereo system—the gift of a grateful member who had saved $80 on a repair that the co-op performed.)

A second co-op organization, the Briarpatch Cooperative Auto Shop Inc., in Palo Alto, Calif., started in much the same way in 1973. It, too, lacked necessary equipment in its early months. But Briarpatch was lucky enough to win a $2,000 foundation grant. And by November 1976 it had eighteen hundred members, each of whom paid $15 to join. Thus, that co-op has been able to buy much of the equipment that the co-op in West Nyack still lacks.

The labor rate at Briarpatch is $17.50 an hour, low for the area. As an alternative, members can rent a stall for $2 an hour or $15 a day and use the shop's tools to perform repairs themselves. (The West Nyack co-op has a similar option, for $3 an hour.) The mechanics will even give members free advice if it doesn't require too much time. Briarpatch gives a 10 percent discount on parts; members may supply their own parts, if they wish.

The staff includes the equivalent of three and a half mechanics, a mechanic's helper, a parts manager, and a part-time accountant. Mechanics' salaries range from $650 to $950 a month, depending on the employe's financial need.

There's a grievance committee—but it hasn't convened in a year. The mechanics themselves have voted to resolve the most recent complaints in the members' favor. In its third year, Briarpatch for the first time is operating at a slight profit.

In principle, the auto-repair co-op is a fine idea. It offers the likelihood of honest work, the possibility of lower prices, and a feeling that the customer is a participant rather than a victim.

Do it yourself?

Since choosing an auto mechanic is at best a gamble, many car owners probably have wondered whether they could perform some auto maintenance and repairs themselves. We believe many can.

When you do it yourself you may save money. Perhaps just as important, after learning the basics of how a car operates you don't feel at a loss if your car breaks down on the road. You may be able to make an on-the-spot repair that will get you rolling. If not, at least you'll be a little more confident the next time you have to deal with a strange garage.

The ideal way to learn to repair cars is from an expert—either in an adult education course or informally from a friend or relative who's a mechanic. An alternative is to try to learn from a do-it-yourself book—no easy task, in CU's experience. Each of the seven books reviewed below has weaknesses, but we do feel we can recommend the first four. Your choice among those four should depend on how mechanically inclined you are and on how deeply you want to become involved in do-it-yourself automobile work. Sometimes, do-it-yourself books differ in details, such as frequency of oil changes, from the recommendations in the manual and maintenance books that come with the car. Our advice: Always follow the car manufacturer's recommendations.

Basic Automotive Troubleshooting. *By Richard Bean. 144 pages plus fold-out diagrams, paperback. Petersen Publishing Co., $2.95.* This is a down-to-earth, rather well-written book. Its primary purpose is to teach the reader to find the cause of a particular problem, and for many car owners this will be a useful book to read. The weakness of the book is that the basic maintenance jobs and repair procedures are described sketchily when they're described at all. In one section of the book, for example, there is an explanation of how to check the starter motor. If the tests indicate an internal problem, the manual wisely urges the reader to take the starter motor to a professional mechanic for repair. But it does not tell how to remove the starter. Another example: To perform several of the tests in the book, it is necessary to remove the spark plugs. But there is no warning for the beginner that the leads must be replaced in proper order or that it is important that the plugs not be overtightened when replaced.

Some auto problems, however, are so elementary that once they are discovered no repair instructions are necessary. For example, when an engine won't run, the manual advises the reader to check first for an empty fuel tank. Don't laugh—sometimes a defective fuel gauge reads "full" even when the tank is empty. This book tells how to check.

Overall, we agree with the author's basic advice: Before resorting to extensive tearing down, check related components in a logical sequence, starting with the easiest tests and with the components that are most likely to fail. The author concludes that most troubles are minor—and complicated ones should be left to a professional mechanic.

This manual contains lots of large, simple, extremely clear drawings that should help even a novice find the proper part in an automobile engine or chassis.

Basic Auto Repair Manual. *384 pages, paperback. Petersen Publishing Co., $3.95.* This manual, revised annually, is the best we have seen for motorists who have at least a smattering of knowledge about the workings of a car. But even a beginner may benefit from some sections—for example, those on changing engine oil and on maintaining tires.

The manual assumes that the reader is serious enough about maintenance and repair to accumulate a few hundred dollars' worth of special tools and equipment. (The first chapter states that $50 worth of hand tools should be sufficient for 90 percent of the repairs—but the jobs described in the following pages involve far more equipment.)

The book proceeds in an orderly, logical fashion from one system to another. But the beginner would do well to skip the discussion of jobs that many a seasoned mechanic might hesitate to tackle—for example, completely overhauling the engine (even grinding the crankshaft), rebuilding an automatic transmission, or repairing body damage.

The quality of the photos and illustrations varies from very good to very bad, but the writing is informal and generally lucid. Useful features include tune-up specifications for late domestic models and an extensive troubleshooting section outlining problems and cures.

Automotive Tune-Ups for Beginners. *By I. G. Edmonds. 184 pages, hardcover. Macrae Smith Co., $6.50.* This book deals strictly with tuning an engine—and therein lie both its strength and its weakness. Because the book devotes so many pages to so limited a subject, it can (and generally does) cover the subject extremely thoroughly, in simple, easy-to-understand language. However, the home mechanic who wants to burrow deeper into the engine or to service other automotive components must look elsewhere.

The book starts off with one of the clearest descriptions we have seen of how an engine operates. No frills. Just the basics—which is all that a beginner really needs to get started. The second chapter stresses safe working procedures, a subject that is insufficiently emphasized in many repair manuals. Succeeding chapters cover the battery, coil, distributor, spark plugs, timing, and the fuel system —each separately, rather than lumped together. The chapter on emission-control devices is thin—but that may be just as well, since most such devices are best left for professional mechanics to service. The glossary and index are helpful.

The Time-Life Book of the Family Car. *357 pages, hardcover. Time-Life Books, $15.* This is a vast book that attempts to tell the reader all there is to know about cars. Some information is interesting but not utilitarian—sections on the history of the horseless carriage, a spread on antique cars, and a chapter predicting what the transportation of the future will be.

Much of the information on buying a new or used car will be familiar to readers of CONSUMER REPORTS. In some chapters, the authors relentlessly parade a procession of fictional characters to illustrate their points. There's Bill, a thirty-year-old engineer who covets a *Belchfire Brougham;* wife Ann, who drives an aging *Behemoth Eight;* Florence the teacher; Harry the accountant; Lester the businessman; etc. However, the 126 pages devoted to upkeep, maintenance and repairs, tuning, and troubleshooting are especially easy to understand and well illustrated. A glossary and an index are included.

Fixing Cars: A Peoples Primer. *By Rick Greenspan et al. 191 pages, paperback. The San Francisco Institute of Automotive Ecology, $5.* This is surely the most amusing repair manual we have seen. It abounds in folksy anecdotes and off-beat cartoon strips. However, the illustrations sometimes obscure the message being conveyed. And if your car refuses to start in the morning, we wonder whether you'd want to wade through a lot of banter while looking for useful instructions.

The chapter describing how a car works is perhaps more detailed than necessary for most beginners. The chapters on tools and on buying parts are concise and straightforward. Some of the maintenance tips are clear; others, such as the cartoon strip explaining how to check a battery, are oversimplified to the point of uselessness. We don't agree with all of the advice. For example, the manual tells the reader to reline the brakes when they begin to scrape. By that time, chances are that the drums or discs will have been damaged. But on balance, the manual is useful, and certainly not dry. An index is included.

Money-Savers' Do-It-Yourself Car Repair. *By LeRoi Smith. 408 pages, hardcover. Macmillan Publishing Co., Inc., $11.* This is a curious book; its author can't seem to make up his mind about who his audience is.

The organization of the book is hopelessly bad. The first chapter plunges into complete disassembly of the suspension system; anyone capable of such a job has no need for a do-it-yourself primer. Later there's a section entitled "Diagnosing 'Funny Noises,'" which explains that an apparent engine noise might actually be a loose pop bottle inside the door—a bit insulting to one's intelligence.

The book lacks information on tools and equipment. And it assumes that the reader is qualified to remove a steering-gear assembly while at the same time being mystified by the difference between bias-ply and radial-ply tires. The author devotes an entire chapter—eighteen pages—to the workings of the rotary engine. But there are only a couple of pages on the removal of a conventional engine from a car.

We disagree with many of the author's statements—for example, his implication that a bubble-type static wheel balancer is adequate for balancing wheel rims narrower than seven inches.

A Woman's Guide to Fixing the Car. *By Arleen and Paul Weissler. 191 pages. Walker and Co., $6.95 hardcover, $3.95 paperback.* This book claims to make the point that a woman, to be truly liberated, must know how a car works. But the book, like its title, is condescending ("An automobile has a lot of this-connects-to-this-which-connects-to-that about it . . .").

The book doesn't claim to teach its readers how to fix something—only to help them understand what needs to be fixed so they can deal intelligently with mechanics. In that case, the authors have devoted far more space than necessary to the intricacies of how a car works.

Many statements in the book are suspect or downright wrong. The authors maintain that when the ammeter or warning light indicates that the generator is discharging, one might drive on for as long as two hours. But if the cause of the discharging is a broken fan belt, even if the battery could hold out that long, the engine might not. Without the fan belt, the water pump in some cars is disabled—and the engine would overheat within minutes. The book maintains that when the clutch starts to slip, its friction disc must be replaced. But often, a simple clutch adjustment is all that's needed—at a saving of $150 to $200. And a grinding noise during shifting doesn't necessarily mean that the transmission must be overhauled, as the book maintains. Again, adjusting the clutch or shift linkage may be the answer. The authors warn that holes in the exhaust system produce "loud noises." But such holes can also produce dead people if the exhaust gases find their way inside the car.

How to Shop
for a Summer Camp

Choosing a summer camp, like choosing a school or college,
bears little resemblance to most product-buying decisions.
The product—part pleasure and part education—can't be examined in a store or tested in a laboratory like a washing
machine. Yet parents who are facing the need to choose a
summer camp for the first time and who wish to make as
intelligent a choice as possible need not rely solely on their
intuition—nor on four-color brochures or slide shows ea-
gerly presented by camp directors. There is a more rational
approach parents can take to the selection process. To buttress our research on that question, CU enlisted the help of
CONSUMER REPORTS readers who had been through the
camp-selection process. From their answers to a detailed
questionnaire* and from interviews with consultants in the

*Our survey was taken following the summer of 1974. We received
close to eleven hundred reports from parents, counselors, counselors-
in-training, and campers. The responses were not particularized for
a specific year and remain valid.

field, we have developed guidelines that should give you a good chance of finding the right camp for your child.

The selection process involves three basic steps: deciding what kind of camp you (and your child) want, locating a group of camps that meet that description, and choosing a camp from that group.

What Kind of Camp

Once exposed to the wide world of camping, you'll find that there are many preliminary decisions you can (and must) make to reduce the number of choices.

How much can you spend? Scout and Camp Fire camps typically cost between $35 and $60 a week for a one-or-two-week summer session. "Y" camps or camps sponsored by religious organizations may run $50 to $85 a week. Private camps cluster in the $120-to-$160 -a-week range for seasons of four or eight weeks. Specialized camps, such as those emphasizing reading, weight loss, or foreign languages, will generally cost slightly more than a regular program.

In our survey, the percentage of campers who said they had a good time was no higher at the most expensive camps than at the cheapest. That could mean that there's no significant relationship between the cost of a camp and satisfaction with it—or it could mean that there are lower expectations at less expensive camps.

How long a camp session do you want? Camp stays come in many lengths, usually from one week to eight weeks. Camps that offer an eight-week session will often agree to let you contract for either half of that time.

What do you expect from the camp experience? Parents and campers should make a list of goals. These might include specific skills to be learned or practiced (snorkeling, reading, music), desirable activities (overnight camping trips, canoeing, competitive sports), or a particular type of organization (highly scheduled days with many required activities, or, conversely, unscheduled days with time to relax and freedom to choose one's activities).

Unless parents and campers agree on goals, one or the other may be unhappy with the camp experience. One mother told us she was disheartened because her eleven-year-old son preferred not to take swimming and he was not required to ("the atmosphere was *very* free"). The camper, however, said he had a great time, especially at arts and crafts. Another family reported that their extremely active son did well at a private camp—"the result of our search for a camp that required the camper to sign up for an activity each period."

Do you want a general or specialty camp? Most youngsters, particularly those not yet in their teens, are probably best off with a varied program. Some specialty camps—basketball, baseball, tennis, sailing—are more school or clinic than camp. But our survey showed that most parents of children who had gone to such specialty camps seemed to be satisfied with the balance between the specialty and other camp activities. And almost half of them said their youngsters had benefited even more than expected from the specialty program. If no more than three hours a day are devoted to the special activity, there's usually ample time for a good mix of other activities.

Do you want a coed camp? A child psychiatrist and a family therapist, in separate interviews, recommended camps where boys and girls share most activities as a healthier selection for children of all ages than sex-segregated camps. If you feel strongly about encouraging or discouraging competitiveness, note that CU's survey indicates that all-boy camps are most likely to be competitive, with coed camps next most likely.

How much creature comfort? Camps range from very comfortable on down—way, way down. First-time campers should be made aware that camp life may mean not only no television, but no hot water, no flush toilets, and no screens between camper and mosquitoes. (Quite a few campers noted with disfavor the lack of flush toilets.)

What size camp do you want? Our survey didn't turn up any relationship between the size of a camp and the overall quality of the camping experience. Most parents in CU's survey thought that camp staffs gave their children enough individual attention, no matter what the size of the camps. (But there was a distinct relationship between the parents' judgment of "enough" attention and the *cost* of the camp. A higher percentage of camps that cost less than $100 a week in 1974 were rated fair or poor on individual attention than were more expensive camps.)

Finding Suitable Camps

Once you have made these preliminary decisions, you will have to find camps that fit the criteria you've developed. There are many sources for leads to camps, but unfortunately none good enough to rely on without further checking. Camp directories, described on pages 358-363, can help you start sorting out camps that seem worth investigating.

There is no such thing as a thoroughly reliable camp accreditation program. Current accreditation by the American Camping Association (ACA) is the most meaningful single credential a camp can offer. But even ACA criteria necessarily omit important subjective factors, and the on-site inspection on which the accreditation is based can be as much as five years old (by 1979 the maximum time between ACA inspection visits is to be three years).

In 1976, 30 percent of the camps checked by the ACA failed to meet the association's standards. Absence of accreditation by the ACA, however, can also mean simply that a camp does not choose to affiliate with the organization. Some camps meet all ACA standards but never apply for ACA accreditation. And, of course, some camps don't want to go to the effort and expense of meeting minimum ACA standards.

There are also professional camp referral services (listed in the Yellow Pages under "Camps"). These services earn commissions from the camps they refer you to. Regard them only as a convenient first source of the kind of information the camp itself would give, not as an objective third party. Much more valuable are the evaluations of families that have had direct experience with a particular camp. Parents of other children you know are a good place to start. But, of course, your children's needs may be quite different from those of your neighbors' children, so you cannot let the choice rest solely on their recommendations.

Some localities have already developed resources you can tap. For example, the Parents League of New York keeps a file of children's and parents' evaluations of summer camps and other summer experiences; members may use the file and an advisory service. The Parents League of New York and the similar Boston Parents League serve parents of children in private schools, but some public schools have developed such share-the-experience systems. And you could join with other parents to compile one.

You don't have much of a choice among Boy Scout camps since most boys go with their own troops, usually to one of the camps owned by the local Boy Scouts of America Council. The camps may vary appreciably in quality. Regional teams inspect each of the six hundred camps of the Boy Scouts of America each year, usually in the first week of operation, and assign a Class A, B, or C rating the same day. All camps must meet basic health, safety, and sanitation standards. Class A camps (a little more than half of all Scout camps) meet all of the 118 camp standards of Boy Scouts of America. B and C ratings usually result from specific deficiencies in program or staff. To find out last year's rating of the camp your boy's troop would attend, call the local B.S.A. Director of Camping. Ask for both the initial and the final rating (camps can be upgraded during the season if they come into compliance with more standards).

The Girl Scouts and Camp Fire Girls run their own camps (see pages 361-362). They typically give you more of a choice than the Boy Scouts.

Making a Choice

After you've narrowed your choice to a few camps that might meet your needs, it's time to talk with their directors. Owner-directors of private camps often visit homes of prospective campers in metropolitan areas or arrange for family appointments in a central location. Distant private camps often accept collect calls from potential customers. You may not be able to talk with the director of a nonprofit camp, such as a Scout or "Y" camp. But do seek information from representatives of the sponsoring agency.

Here's a list of key questions to ask a camp director and some guides to interpreting the answers.

What is the director's age and background? According to ACA criteria, camp directors should be at least twenty-five years old, should hold at least a Bachelor's degree, and should have had at least two summers of administrative or supervisory experience in a camp. That seems pretty minimal, though. You may well want more maturity and experience than that.

How long has the director run the camp? "Camp Wonderwood—since 1925" and all of Camp Wonderwood's distinguished past mean very little if the current director took over only two months ago. When inquiring about a camp, ask how long and in what capacity the director has been associated with that camp. Ask for the same information concerning the camps with which the director was previously associated.

What does the director do off-season and what is the director's permanent address? Check out what you're told. One parent told us about a director who misrepresented his off-season employment. Any misrepresentation should make you sufficiently suspicious to cross that camp off your list. **Does the director live at the camp during the season?** You want to be assured that the director indeed directs—is personally visible, personally involved with the program and people. You might also find out if the director eats in the dining hall with the campers. If camp food isn't good enough for the director, it might not be good enough for your child.

What are the camp's goals? What interests and hobbies are encouraged at the camp? How would the director describe the ideal camper? Ask these questions before mentioning your own expectations or discussing your child's virtues or foibles. Otherwise, you might encounter a director with a flexible philosophy whose chief interest is in attracting paying campers. Competent directors will ask leading questions of their own about your child and will honestly tell you if they think your child won't be happy at the camp. Listen with the "third ear." An effective director ought to show enthusiasm for the camp's philosophy and program. On the other hand, missionary zeal (for or against competitive sports, for example) may indicate a view quite different from your own.

What is the policy on visits and phone calls? The policy and the reasons given for it may well tell you a great deal about the style of the camp. An easygoing camp might welcome visitors at any time as proof that the atmosphere is not "dressed up" for visiting day. But so permissive a policy might tend to disrupt the program and make it harder for campers to focus on camp instead of home. At the other extreme, a camp that virtually forbids such contacts is rigid indeed. You'll want assurances that your child will not be a prisoner.

Are children encouraged to write home? Both children and parents can have separation anxiety. As a parent, you may be very glad to get a letter, even if it just says: "Sam said everybody has to write home before we can go swimming. How are you? I am fine." Many camps see to it that children write home once a week.

What facilities does the camp have and where are they? Confirm the existence and condition of basic facilities. Get details on special facilities that are important to your camper. If swimming is a high-priority activity, for example, find out the dimensions of the pool, whether that picturesque lake can be used for swimming, how much of the day can be devoted to swimming and swimming instruction, how many pairs of water skis and how many motorboats to pull water-skiers are available. Be sure to find out where the promised activities will take place. A parent who sent her child to a Florida baseball school told us that a key facility—the baseball playing fields—was several miles from the camp.

What is the schedule like? Listen for evidence of where the camp falls in the range between highly structured activity and unpressured drifting. Be sure to pinpoint how electives, trips, and workshops are assigned. In some camps, younger or less aggressive campers never get a chance at the popular electives. Other camps tie youngsters down to early choices even if the choices turn out to be disappointing.

What happens when bad weather interferes with the regular program? Listen for a list of specific strategies, not just general assurances. The director should have planned activities that can fill many active hours and have on hand materials for those activities. Such indoor projects as working on sets and costumes for a play outscore writing letters home and playing checkers, or even watching movies, a rainy-day equivalent of television at home. It's helpful if there is a large indoor space on the campsite—or at least one available and contracted for nearby. This can be a key question, for in our survey 44 percent of parents and 72 percent of counselors rated their camp as poor or only fair on rainy-day activities. Parent-staff communications was the only other factor rated so low by anywhere near so many respondents.

Is the camp coed? What activities are shared? If you want a sex-integrated experience for your child, be sure the camp is really coed and not just next door to a brother or sister camp. Living quarters should be in the same area, and most activities should be shared, giving boys and girls natural opportunities for casual friendships.

What is the ratio of counselors to campers? ACA standards prescribe at least one counselor for every five children six years old or under; one counselor for every six campers the ages of seven and eight; one for every eight campers between the ages of nine and fourteen. There's too much penny-pinching on staff if your child is not under the care of both the bunk counselor and a qualified waterfront staff when swimming, or if counselors don't seem to get a child-free break for two hours each day. (Counselors with battle fatigue can't give your child their best.) A general counselor who also served as swimming instructor told CU that there was understaffing "because in the daytime they also brought in day campers, which doubled the number of children to take care of."

How are counselors recruited? Competent directors find and keep competent staff. A good camp will have most slots filled by returning staffers. Specialists should have extensive credentials—not just a one-week crash course. ACA standards specify that at least 80 percent of the counselors and program staff should be eighteen or older and that at least 20 percent of the program and administrative staff should be college graduates.

How does the camp prepare staff members for their responsibilities? A good camp will have a planned orientation program for staff, including at least five days of pre-camp training on the campsite and regular staff meetings during the season to increase competency in dealing with program problems and camper problems.

Who prepares the meals? Meals may be prepared in camp by a separate food staff. Or some or all food may be brought in by an institutional purveyor (often a nearby college with unused summer food-service capacity) or by a commercial firm of the kind that provision many employe cafeterias. That's not necessarily bad, but the food delivered will not be the farm-fresh country-kitchen meals you may automatically associate with camp. Children should be allowed seconds on main courses.

Is there comprehensive liability insurance? The camp should have comprehensive liability insurance and you should understand exactly which types of accidents are covered by the camp's policy and which are not.

What are the arrangements for medical care? Campers should be required to submit a medical report ahead of time. If they are not, they should be examined on arrival at camp. Health records, including a camp record of accidents, first aid, and medical treatment, should be on file. Pertinent medical information should be shared with the staff. One counselor told us of a child with an ulcer problem unknown to the staff until the girl became ill.

If there's no resident physician or registered nurse, there should be a firm understanding between the camp and one or more local physicians for medical services in case of illness or injury. If you want to be informed of every ailment or accident, even a minor one, be sure the director understands and agrees. One parent told CU she learned her son had had overnight medical care for sunburn and heat exposure only when he told her about it after the season.

What are the sleeping arrangements? Sleeping quarters should provide cross-ventilation. There should be at least six feet between the heads of sleepers and at least thirty inches between the sides of beds. Campers' sleeping accommodations should not be isolated from supervisors'. There should be fire-detecting equipment and fire escapes in rooms above ground level.

What are toilet and shower facilities like? Your camper should know in advance how primitive the living conditions will be. The condition of the toilet facilities dismayed a number of the campers who responded to CU's survey. More than 25 percent of the counselors said their camp did not have enough showers for the campers. ACA recommends a minimum of one shower head for twenty persons; some states now require one shower head for every ten persons.

How are campers transported during the season? Many camps transport youngsters in unsafe, open-bed trucks; be sure your child will ride seated in an enclosed vehicle. More than 15 percent of respondent counselors reported unsafe vehicles at their camps; 5 percent reported unlicensed drivers.

What are the swimming arrangements? A swimming area in shallow water should be roped off for those who are learning to swim. All swimmers should be safely separated from boating and water-skiing areas. You should sense enthusiasm for a strictly enforced buddy system. Ask about supervision. According to ACA standards, it is "highly recommended" that the waterfront supervisor be at least twenty-one years old. The supervisor should hold a current Red Cross Water Safety Instructor certificate or an equivalent "Y" or Scout certificate. There should be enough qualified aquatic counselors (with lifesaving certificates) to provide at least one qualified counselor for every ten campers in the water.

How are campers supervised on trips and on travel outside the basic camp? There should always be a qualified leader in charge of trip programs. The leader should be someone with basic training in first aid and in rescue methods. Trip equipment should include ample first aid material in case of emergencies.

What does the fee cover? Many camps charge a fee that covers most or all of these items: registration, infirmary, insurance, trips away from camp, craft materials. More than 40 percent of CU respondents paid in excess of $25 in extras, including canteen (money parents put into a spending fund for their children to cover expenses not included in the camping fee) ; 26 percent paid more than $50. Ten percent of the families paid unexpected extra charges; in half the cases, these totaled $50 or more.

It's usual to make a canteen deposit against which the camper draws. Be sure that limits are enforced, that accounts will be presented to you, and that leftover canteen money will be returned at the season's end.

Be sure that the contract description of what is covered by the fee does not contradict information you may have received from the camp representative.

What about tipping? The director should take a firm position against tipping. Tipping suggests that differential treatment of campers is possible. The ACA standards call for a written rule discouraging it (which may explain why we were told of a camp where the director discouraged tipping in public and encouraged it at camp). Only 3 percent of the parents in CU's survey reported that they tipped counselors or promised them a tip at the beginning of the camping session.

Is there a rebate if the camper leaves early? Only 3 percent of the children in CU's survey did not stay for the term contracted for. But should your child be one of those who must leave camp because of illness, injury, or preference, you could lose a good deal of money if there is no rebate provision clearly stated in the contract.

Will the director give references—names, addresses, and phone numbers of some former campers and counselors in your general area? A list of a dozen names (or a camp yearbook giving everyone's name) is more useful than just one or two names, which the director may have carefully preselected.

When you discuss the camp with former campers and their parents, you should have two aims in mind. The first will be to confirm the specifics already given to you by the camp director—such as the ratio of counselors to campers, the number of campers in a bunk, the provisions for rainy-day activities, and so on. The second, and perhaps more important, aim will be to get as forthright an assessment of the camp as possible from the parents' (and/or camper's) point of view. The key question here is whether the camper wants to return—and whether the parents would send him or her. Returning is the sincerest form of appreciation; 65 percent of parents in our survey who had previously sent children to camp returned a child to the same camp.

In addition, part of the test should be the question of whether the director or other camp representative holds still for so many questions. Our camp consultant, in her role as parent, ran through all the CU questions and more in phone calls with two directors. The evasive and querulous answers of one director were as enlightening as the prompt and detailed replies of the other.

Safety: Government Gets Involved

Parents tend to assume that summer camps, like schools, operate in compliance with some legal requirements about staff qualifications and safety of buildings and program activities. Often, that's not so. Very few states require any special training for counselors who supervise such activities as water sports, riflery, and horseback riding. As of 1976, thirty-four states had no regulations on personnel, thirteen states had none on program safety, and six states had none on health and medical services. In addition, thirty-nine states had no regulations on transportation and thirty-six had none regarding out-of-camp trips and primitive outpost camps. Five states had no regulations on sanitation and food or on camp site and facilities.

Only eleven states have comprehensive youth camp safety regulations that are effective and functioning. Eight of these states—California, Colorado, Connecticut, Illinois, Kentucky, Michigan, New York, and Texas—administer camp regulations through a centralized state office. (New Jersey has enacted a comprehensive set of safety regulations, but the program is not yet fully implemented.) The other three states—Maine, New Hampshire, and Vermont—have decentralized camp supervision, involving a variety of state agencies.

The Youth Camp Safety Act was designed to get the remaining states to take action by providing a carrot—federal money—and a stick—federal intervention. Passed by the House of Representatives in April 1975, the bill never reached the Senate floor for a vote. Two members of Congress from Connecticut, Ronald Sarasin and Stewart McKinney, plan to introduce substantially the same legislation in 1977.

The version passed by the House in 1975 would have established an Office of Youth Camp Safety within the Department of Health, Education, and Welfare (HEW). That office would be charged with developing comprehensive youth camp safety standards within a reasonable time after the effective date of the bill. States would then have to develop, and win HEW approval of, their own standards, which must be "at least as effective" as HEW standards. Camps in states that failed to do so would be subject to federal regulation and enforcement. When federal inspection turned up substandard conditions, camps would be counseled on how to correct them and given time to do so. Only repeated or willful violations would be punished by revocation of license or by civil fines. States would be eligible to receive federal money, which could be used to cover much of a state's costs in developing and implementing standards.

No matter what eventually comes out of Congress, it will take active consumers in every state to see that state-developed plans are good ones and that they are fully implemented.

A Review of Camp Directories

There are a number of camp directories that may help you match a camp to the criteria you've developed. Some of the more widely available directories and lists are described below, in order of estimated usefulness. Since the bare fact that a given camp exists may be what you most need to know, we recommend that you also check for compilations that may be put out by parent groups, social service organizations (camps for handicapped or disadvantaged), religious groups, fraternal organizations, and other such organizations.

Parents' Guide to Accredited Camps (separate editions for each of four regions: Northeastern, Southern, Midwestern, and Western), American Camping Association, Bradford Woods, Martinsville, Ind. 46151. Each paperback guide is $1.95 plus 45 cents postage/handling and can be ordered through one of the ACA's thirty-four sectional headquarters or from the main office in Indiana. (Be sure to indicate which of the four editions you wish to order.) Editions range in size from ninety-six pages (Northeastern, which describes about twelve hundred camps) to forty-eight pages (Southern, which describes about five hundred camps). Included in the four editions are all of the ACA camps accredited as of November 1, 1976. The guides give comprehensive factual information about each camp included: camp name, type, director, operator, winter and summer addresses, enrollment capacity, length of sessions, rates, aquatic facilities, housing facilities, clientele (disadvantaged, intercultural, etc.), ages, sex. An index lists camps by specialty: music, backpacking, religious emphasis, etc. Accredited camps meet fourteen mandatory standards and at least 80 percent of the many additional standards on safety, program, personnel, administration, and site. ACA-trained "certified visitors" make on-site accreditation inspections while camp is in session. Note that ACA lists only paid-up ACA-affiliated camps and that inspections can have taken place as much as five years ago. Each edition includes a section advising parents on how to shop for a summer camp. There are also paid advertisements from some of the camps that are listed in the four editions of the guide.

Porter Sargent Guide to Summer Camps and Summer Schools, 1975-76, Porter Sargent Publishers, Inc., 11 Beacon St., Boston, Mass. 02108. 480 pages, paperback, $5; hardcover, $8. The nineteenth edition of this biennial camping guide lists some eleven hundred camps and schools. A seventy-page section of paid advertisements for camps and schools precedes the "Descriptive Listing." The listing itself is a compilation of "information supplied by administrators in response to questionnaires and correspondence." Inclusion of a camp does not imply compliance with any group of standards. A typical listing gives basic data including, for example, type of housing and whether a camp has a counselor-in-training program. Evaluative comments ("relevant and exciting"), where they appear, are provided by the camps themselves.

How to Select a Private Camp for Your Child, 1976 directory of Association of Private Camps, 55 West 42 St., New York, N.Y. 10036. 48-page booklet, free. This booklet gives basic factual information about some one hundred member-camps concentrated in the Northeast. Housing is not routinely described. Puffery statements supplied by camps, such as "superior facilities," are included. The Association of Private Camps says camps listed affirm adherence to APC standards and most camps have also been evaluated by an APC team or a professional evaluator.

Directory of Jewish Resident Summer Camps, National Jewish Welfare Board, 15 East 26 St., New York, N.Y. 10010. 100 pages, $3. Listings for 270 camps give capacity, age groups, sex, summer and winter addresses, name of director, how many sessions, rates, and dietary practice. Camps listed are operated "under the auspices of" the National Jewish Welfare Board, Jewish community centers,

YM and YWHAs, B'nai B'riths, ideological movements, synagogues, or other Jewish communal organizations. "Listing of a camp in this Directory in no way implies an endorsement or approval of the camp or its program by the National Jewish Welfare Board. . . . Information . . . was furnished by the operating organization."

YMCA Directory of Resident Camping, 1976-77, National Board of YMCAs, Urban Action and Program Division, 291 Broadway, New York, N.Y. 10007. 68 pages, $1.50. This booklet lists sponsoring "Y," camp name, winter and summer addresses, camp director, age range and sex of campers (increasingly, "Y" camps are coed), approximate daily summer fee; it does not describe programs. Write sponsoring "Y" for program information and other details. National organization sets standards, which are correlated with ACA standards.

YWCA. For information about YWCA resident camps, write to Data Center, YWCA National Board, 600 Lexington Ave., New York, N.Y. 10022. The Data Center will refer inquiries to the appropriate national office in one of the four regions. That national office, in turn, will suggest which community association you can write to for detailed information about a YW camp. There are at present eighty-one YW camps, which serve girls and women only. The national organization does not set standards.

1976 Directory Issue of Canadian Camping Magazine, Canadian Camping Association, 102 Eglinton Ave. East, Toronto, Ont. M4P1E1. 75 pages of the issue are devoted to the directory; $1.50. This directory lists more than five hundred resident camps accredited by the Canadian Camping Association. Gives name and location, date founded, winter address, capacity, sessions, fee, camp's statement of purpose. Beginning in 1977, each of the provinces will publish its own camping directory. The national organization has developed uniform standards for camps. Accrediting is done by the provincial association. According to the Ontario Camping Association, teams do site visits every three or four years.

Girl Scouts. Individual directory lists for each of six regions available from Girl Scouts of the U.S.A., Recruitment and Referral Section, Human Resources Dept., 830 Third Ave., New York, N.Y. 10022. Various formats; typically several pages each. Free. Most directories give basic information about the resident camps and troop camp sites in a region: location, capacity, age range, special emphases (marine biology, horseback riding, sailing, primitive camping, etc.). Some also note natural features (lake, pond, woods), indicate which camps have ACA accreditation, which camps accept campers from outside the local council. Name and address of the local council that operates a given camp are listed; the local council must be contacted for information on current fees, program details, etc. Girl Scouts of the U.S.A. has developed a list of "recognized and desirable standards" for camps. Resident camps are visited periodically by members of national staff or regional board who fill out a camp-appraisal form. A camp that cannot meet minimum safety standards can be closed down. Many Girl Scout resident camps are ACA-accredited.

Camp Fire Girls. Persons who wish information about the Camp Fire resident camps—there are two hundred of them —should write, indicating which parts of the country or which specialties (riding, backpacking, etc.) they are interested in. They will be put in touch with local councils that operate such camps. A stamped, self-addressed envelope should accompany each inquiry. Write to Resident Camps, Camp Fire Girls, Inc., 3821 Woodrow Ave., Wichita, Kan. 67204. Camp Fire Girls has developed its own standards for camps and says that they are "equal to and in some respects more stringent than ACA standards." Local councils use Camp Fire Girls standards as guidelines for an annual self-evaluation and report to national headquarters. Site visits by national volunteer and professional staff take place at intervals of one to five years or more. The right to use the Camp Fire Girls name is withdrawn if the Camp Fire Girls program is not being followed, or if there is an imminent threat to health or safety.

Other. In addition to the sources listed above, there are many citywide or regionwide camp lists. For example, United Way in Los Angeles publishes a forty-eight-page booklet bringing together information on more than 125 organization and private resident camps in Southern California. The New York State Camp Directors Association publishes an annual listing of its hundred or so member camps. (To get a copy, send 50 cents to the NYSCDA, Box 364, Lenox Hill Station, New York, N.Y. 10021.) United Camps, Conferences & Retreats puts out a six-page folder with detailed information about camps associated with Presbyterian, United Methodist, and Reformed churches in metropolitan New York. The twenty-four-page directory of the Western Association of Independent Camps gives details on forty-seven resident camps, all ACA-accredited, most in California, some in Arizona, Utah, and Washington. Catholic News, 68 W. Broad St., Mount Vernon, N.Y. 10552, publishes a guide to Catholic camps in New York and other areas of the Northeast. The eight-hundred-camp directory of Christian Camping International is an example of an extensive directory that is not basically intended for the public but that could probably be consulted at one of the thousands of churches to which it is distributed.

Index